CARRIED BY A PROMISE

CARRIED BY A PROMISE
A Life Transformed Through Yoga

SWAMI RADHANANDA

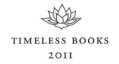

TIMELESS BOOKS
2011

timeless books
www.timeless.org

in Canada:
P.O. Box 9, Kootenay Bay, BC, VOB 1X0
contact@timeless.org
(800) 661-8711

in the United States:
P.O. Box 3543, Spokane, WA, 99220-3543
info@timeless.org
(800) 251-9273

Design by Todd Stewart
Cover photo of Swami Radhananda at Yasodhara Ashram, 1981, courtesy of the author
Author photo by Daniel Seguin

Library and Archives Canada Cataloguing in Publication

Radhananda, Swami, 1941–
    Carried by a promise : a life transformed through yoga / Swami Radhananda.

ISBN 978-1-932018-36-3

    1. Radhananda, Swami, 1941– —Relations with gurus. 2. Radha, Swami
Sivananda, 1911–1995. 3. Yoga. 4. Spiritual life—Hinduism.
5. Gurus—Biography. 6. Spiritual biography—British Columbia. I. Title.

BL73.R34A3 2011   204'.36092   C2010-907153-0

Printed in Canada
Interior: 100% post-consumer-waste recycled acid-free paper
Cover: FSC certified 10% post-consumer-waste recycled paper

Environmental Benefits Statement

By using paper made from post-consumer recycled content,
the following resources have been saved.

⬇ trees	💧 water	○ energy	▤ solid waste	☁ greenhouse gases
18	30,890	6	223	764
fully grown	litres	million BTU	kilograms	kilograms

Environmental impact estimates were made using the Environmental Defense Paper Calculator.
For more information visit http://papercalculator.org.

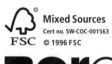

Mixed Sources
Cert no. SW-COC-001563
FSC © 1996 FSC

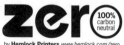

100% carbon neutral

by Hemlock Printers www.hemlock.com/zero

Also by Swami Radhananda

Living the Practice (2011)

Timeless titles by Swami Sivananda Radha

In the Company of the Wise
Time To Be Holy: Collected Satsang Talks
On Sanyas: The Yoga of Renunciation
Light and Vibration
The Yoga of Healing
Kundalini Yoga for the West
Hatha Yoga: The Hidden Language
The Divine Light Invocation
Mantras: Words of Power
When You First Called Me Radha: Poems
The Devi of Speech: The Goddess in Kundalini Yoga
Radha: Diary of a Woman's Search

Timeless titles by other authors

The Inner Life of Asanas by Swami Lalitananda
Inside Outside Overlap by Billy Mavreas
The Glass Seed by Eileen Delehanty Pearkes
Inspired Lives: The Best of Ascent Magazine edited by Clea McDougall
In Durga's Embrace: A Disciple's Diary by Swami Durgananda
Yoga: A Gem for Women by Geeta Iyengar

for Swami Sivananda Radha

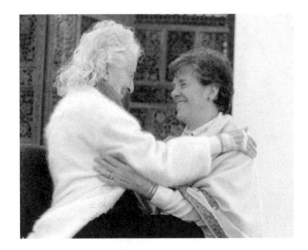

*Swami Radha and Swami Radhananda at the presidential
inauguration, December, 1993. Courtesy of Yasodhara Ashram.*

Table of Contents

Introduction

This book is based on my diaries and follows the thread of my
life from my first meeting with Swami Radha in 1977 until
she died in 1995. A spiritual diary is such an essential part
of learning. By looking back I have recognized the victories,
the difficulties, the mistakes, and the way I learned. I can
also see how the teachings Swami Radha gave me were woven
into my life. Although I worked with her instructions at the
time, it is only now – through reviewing the diaries – that
I recognize more clearly what she was doing and what she
was encouraging me to do. Compiling this memoir was like
looking into a mirror and seeing who I am.

I was deeply attracted to the way Swami Radha taught
and how she opened the space for me to acknowledge the
spiritual dimension of life. Stepping back, I see my life's
patterns – the waves that carry me up and down – but more
importantly, I see the underlying current that is ongoing and
eternal. I truly have been carried by a promise. At any point I
had a choice to get stuck or to keep going and become lighter.
I found that through my devotion to the teachings I was able
to become more who I really am. The work is transforming.

Having a woman as a spiritual teacher was a rare

opportunity. There have always been excellent, intelligent women, but sometimes their methods are not understood. If Swami Radha asked me to make her a cup of tea in a particular way, she wanted to see if I could follow directions in very simple tasks. If I couldn't do it there, how could she ask me to do more? The "more" could be looking after my house or my children or myself effectively and with love. It could be stepping forward to look after a group of people who were searching for what life is about. She had very practical, down-to-earth ways to help me start, and from that foundation she encouraged me to keep going.

Swami Radha supported women and wanted Yasodhara Ashram to be a safe place for women. She gave me the gift of a fulfilling, challenging and inspiring position as her successor. But this path of Light is open to anyone who can honour the Divine Feminine.

Spiritual life isn't easy; it requires stamina and surrender. Spiritual teachers have to be demanding because so few people can make a commitment and stick with it. And there are many illusions about spiritual life. People often think that spiritual is something "beyond," but it really isn't. It is life and what we do with it. At the Ashram we always ask: What is needed now? What is happening in the world? Instead of making linear plans, we follow a more reflective approach – listening for what is needed.

When I first came to the Ashram I wanted my family, my community and my world to become more like the Ashram – more accepting, open and whole. Now, as the world becomes increasingly chaotic and troubled, I see a need to support work that helps eradicate greed and abuse. We need places like the Ashram, where people can feel safe and can sincerely work on themselves. Now is the time to step out of old limitations and to help make the world lighter, clearer and more transparent.

As I write this I see Yasodhara Ashram flourishing,

fulfilling a real need in the world for sacred space, for safe ground to explore life and inner life, to look honestly at where we are and to ask where we are going. As a community we continue to make the Ashram more sustainable for those who will come in the future. As spiritual people this is what we can do: care for the people who are seeking, and do our best to help create a better future.

Looking back over seventeen years of being president of the Ashram, experience has taught me how to make transitions. The Ashram continues to open up. Life and time are saying "succession."

Since the early 1990s we have been inviting in young people through the Teen Program and the Young Adult Program and through work opportunities such as *Ascent* magazine. Now, as we age, the Ashram residents are stepping back and handing over more of the management to the younger people, who are eager to learn. But at the same time we recognize the need for an inner core of people willing to commit and to sacrifice in order to take care of the teachings and this sacred place. Many people have good ideas, but where are all the Radhas? Where are those whose love for the Divine comes first in their lives?

So I hold the space, waiting to see what will come next. I invite people in – into the community, into more responsibility, into more in-depth work on themselves, into the promises that will carry them. I prepare the ground, extend the invitation, and wait.

I have the example of Swami Radha, who trained many people as potential caretakers of the teachings. She knew how to wait, how to listen for the Divine messages, how to read the signs. I feel privileged to have known such an extraordinary teacher and woman, and to have had a lifetime of learning, which continues to this day.

— *Swami Radhananda, fall 2010, Yasodhara Ashram*

The Beginning

Streaming droplets of light shower down on me like crystals, tiny shining bits like heaven's rain. The room becomes very bright, I feel bright, and it turns so silent. Little stars settle in us and around us and I even breathe them in. I open my eyes a crack and see everyone concentrated and glowing. Closing my eyes, it is quiet beyond quietness, bright beyond brightness.

Susan is leading our women's group in a standing meditation. I am amazed at the intimacy of it. We invoke light and it fills us, making itself part of me, the whole space, and everybody in it. The dark, dingy church basement is transformed.

So this is yoga – it must be something extraordinary!

I have been depressed and my best friend, Susan, wants to share what has helped her. In May she attended Ten Days of Yoga at "the Ashram" and she's already taught the Divine

Light Invocation to our women's group. She has also shown me how to work with dreams and chant mantras to calm my mind. I especially like finding the messages in my dreams.

Now we've both signed up for a conference called Women and Spiritual Life, which seems right somehow. Still, I'm nervous. I'm excited but also leery as we arrive at the Ashram. Will it be weird, foreign, full of swamis? What are they? What will they say? How will I fit in?

Stepping out of the VW van onto the ashram ground, I smell something familiar, fresh, uplifting. "I've been here before" – that's the feeling I get from the smell. I don't know how to explain it, but I feel connected and I know I will be safe here and that everything will be fine. Surrounded by trees and greenness, I feel as if I am back in the dream I had last night where I was driving to a hidden place, a familiar place behind the mountain and into a valley, a place that was hard to find and very far from everything else, especially from my family and friends.

The dream lingers as we walk to the office, where a woman comes to greet us. She looks happy and is such a lovely person, so normal. We register and settle in at the Guest Lodge, and then Susan shows me around. We walk down the path past Main House, which is the kitchen and dining room, to the Beach Prayer Room, a little wooden A-frame overlooking the lake. When I open the door – again a wonderful smell – it is familiar, like something I remember.

The next morning we go to our class and sit in a big circle of women. The ashram women are dressed in skirts and nylons and the rest of us look like hippies in old jeans and t-shirts.

"What is it to be a woman?" they ask, and we write our own reflections on these questions. I explore my ideas of wife, mother, daughter, sister, teacher.... As a woman I sometimes feel powerless, dismissible, invisible. I am responsible for nurturing, loving and consoling my children and my husband. At work I am a doer and a problem-solver. I have resisted entering the unknown spiritual part of me and have only seen it through small cracks.

Who am I? How am I changing? I am thirty-six years old and have a feeling I haven't been changing. I am aware that I am a woman, but not beyond, to who I am. I suddenly understand that I don't know who I am. Strange...

For two days we write, we read our responses and talk to each other, we do spiritual practices. Everything goes deep and directs me back to myself and to what I think. I have very powerful feelings. Sometimes I feel frightened or mistrustful at the start of an exercise. Or I imagine something dramatic will happen and then hit a barrier. That same dream I had just before coming here keeps arising in my mind. The building we are in seems just like the long cedar building in my dream. And today I saw the little cabin from my dream where Susan's husband, Russell, was standing on the porch and Susan was wading across the rushing stream. That stream is here too. How could I see something in a dream before I actually experienced it? Why is it all so familiar?

I explore my fear of crisis, of losing things. I remember the last party I went to and how futile it seemed, yet how frightened I am of losing my friends, my marriage.

"Keep a spiritual diary," they say. "Ask yourself questions, observe your feelings. Choose something to work on and write down your insights and intuitions. Review it once a month." I'm going to try this when I get home.

There is an underlying question in my life: Is this it? I have done many of the expected things – gone to school, university, taught school, married, had children, been involved in community projects and women's groups. I'm starting a daycare, something I really believe in. I love my two young children. Still there seems to be something missing. Is this it?

This afternoon Swami Radha comes to speak to us. Something inside me is touched by her wisdom. She looks more like a well-dressed and kindly grandmother than my image of what a swami would be. She appears to be ordinary, but I know she is extraordinary after a moment in her presence. I am struck by the power behind her speech, and the simplicity of the teachings.

After she has spoken to us, all I can say is: Why haven't I heard this before? Why hasn't anyone else said this to me?

She speaks about the purpose of life, living life fully with quality. She talks about the Light. She gives everyday examples that are the essence of simplicity. Swami Radha talks of making times with the family quality time. Mealtimes could be made different by paying special attention to detail in order to appreciate what is received, making the setting and presentation pleasant, and sincerely giving thanks.

She tells a story of her guru pouring cream into the black coffee until the cup is filled with white cream. The blackness is transformed.

And she talks of climbing the snow-peaked mountains to the top and how lonely it is. She encourages women to lift their focus to the Most High, and stop being so immature and selfish. It is a challenge to live life fully and not get stuck at the bottom of the mountain. My heart aches for her and I want to help.

She says that every woman is complete in herself and must allow the completeness to manifest. A woman who wants quality shouldn't be involved with a man who doesn't want quality. What do you want your life to be? If you haven't brought quality into your own life, you can't ask it of others.

Then she speaks of doing the Divine Light Invocation once a day, and life will take on a different meaning. She promises that the effort to cooperate with the evolution of consciousness is worth it. She challenges, "Aren't there women out there who are willing to aspire?"

I can feel part of me wanting to step onto this path, and part of me definitely wanting to stay right in the security of the known pain and darkness. It seems scary and very distant, this message of change and effort.

But I decide I will do one Divine Light Invocation a day. What can I lose?

In the evening we gather for satsang in the Beach Prayer Room and chant *Hari Om* for a long time. Then the swami who is leading gives a talk about Divine Light – light as not being heavy, light as being any form you want it to be. Together we start to repeat the Divine Light mantra: I am created by Divine Light. I am sustained by Divine Light. I am protected by Divine Light. I am surrounded by Divine Light. I am ever growing into Divine Light.

When we say the first line, "I am created by Divine Light," the Light seems to shoot right out of my head and tries to lift me up and out the window. I try to let it go but it holds me, and I feel a strong power in me. As I relax the feeling becomes fine, warm, close. I am astonished, kind of scared and unbelieving. What is happening? It is as though I am being stretched and the space opens for the Light, which is like a white form with the qualities of a warm, kind, loving woman. I feel her Light within me.

When satsang ends I can't move. I start to rub my face and breathe. I feel very strange. I leave with Susan holding me tightly as we both walk up the little path. I will have to keep this to myself. Arthur would not understand. Even I don't understand.

Back in class the next day we are asked to reflect on where we are in our lives. Before moving to Lethbridge my husband and I had been travelers – living at a commune on the Sunshine Coast in BC, then moving to Cambridge, England for Arthur's PhD studies. With the birth of my son, Garth, in 1970 I had an almost immediate realization of my mother – of flesh and bones and a strong tie that holds us together. I suddenly knew that she had done her best, whatever her shortcomings. From Cambridge we went to Mexico for Arthur's anthropology fieldwork. The inclusiveness of the culture impressed me, how people of all ages supported each other and supported me as a mother of a young child. Then we went back to Cambridge and my daughter Clea was born. She will soon be four and as she grows she overwhelms me with her beauty and femininity, so different from me.

When Arthur completed his studies he was offered a job at the University of Lethbridge. We thought we would just stop over for a while and he could finish his thesis. But we decided to settle. For the first time I was doing something I wanted to do. I helped to start a daycare centre – it is a very good one. And I am involved in a women's consciousness-raising group. From being just a mother and a teacher, I have become a thinking person.

We bought an old three-storey house with trees and a garden – but as soon as we did, my husband was not rehired at the university. Did that mean we would have to move and leave everything I had worked so hard for? The day he told me, I was overcome with grief. I sat down and something pulled away from my body. I felt something leave me. I couldn't relate or do anything for days except cry or be angry.

Then I started to do some jogging. I hadn't run since I was twelve years old. It made me aware of my physical being. I joined a yoga class and that made me aware of my mind and body working together. Many areas of my body weren't working – my shoulders wouldn't move, I couldn't bend. They gradually started coming back to life and a space in my mind of quiet and stillness, which I had never used, opened up. So I've been getting up earlier, making space for these practices.

Now that I have found the Ashram it feels as though I have what I need to support the next changes in my life. Looking at where I am at the close of this conference, I would say I want to bring my ideals to life. I want to practise nonattachment, letting go of expectations. I want to open up to the Most High and take a forward direction. I want to give myself time to myself and feed that desire to grow. I want to be able to pay the bills. And I want to keep surrounded by Light.

Fall 1977

When I return home and begin the Light practice I'm not sure if I expect results or maybe just fear change. What will it bring? I worry that everyone will notice that I am different. Slowly I begin to bring little changes into my family life – quality time and actions, time to really connect with the children, to appreciate what I have. Do the Divine Light once a day. At first it feels awkward, but I persist.

I hoped Arthur would be interested, but it is as if he has stopped growing as I have started. He seems to have no ambition to get a job and he isn't working on his thesis at all. I am the one looking after everybody and I want his help. I am committed to our marriage and think I can help him by bringing good things into his life, such as good food and good ideas. I should be able to help him evolve, especially now that I have some tools.

Can I let things go? Will he find his own pace? How do I influence him? What can I do that is directive yet not nagging? Why would a forty-six-year-old man not look after himself? Should I do it? How do I deal with emotions? How should I deal with them?

Things I liked about today – feeling good and putting the kindergarten room into the Light. Doing garden work. Walking home with Garth. Singing Divine Mother and *Om Namah Sivaya*. Working with the children. Things I didn't like – Arthur's aimlessness and drunken and uncared-for behaviour. How can I change? Be more kind to Arthur. Hold Clea more. Breathe deeply and say the mantra when in crisis.

I read over all I had written at the Women and Spiritual Life conference. I find it difficult to be clear. What are my ideals? Who is that white form that I experienced in satsang and where is she now? How often can I receive the Light and use it? What am I supposed to do, exactly? What about mantras? Can I use them for the sake of repeating them because they sound nice? Must I have a purpose? How do I recognize what I need here? How do I know if my actions and reactions are right?

I seem to be under the shadow of a former religious dogma and one that I can't figure out. I don't feel confident. I feel as though I am very young and childish, sometimes embarrassed. Why do I cry for Swami Radha and feel overwhelmed by the Light?

How can I grasp that strength and energy back from the conference? Was it real? Or was it just relaxation and opening? Or brainwashing into a way of life that I won't be able to cope with? Who is writing this anyway?

A busy weekend... I go shopping with Clea, chant mantra in the car, pick veggies, go for a walk in the warm, bright coulees. I find Arthur's energy draining. To do: write letters, give tomatoes to friends, do more yoga, be more accepting. What is spiritual? Sunday: make bread, pick beans, do work for Early Childhood Education certification, make chutney, walk with Clea, make supper, talk to a friend, go to satsang at Susan's, feel elated. I love chanting. Just do actions, confusion will fall away.

At the women's group this week I get a flash when everyone was talking about their weekends, that no one is in control of their lives. We don't know the reason why we do things. We don't question enough, we just accept. What has happened to us as women that we can't see why we are here, where we are going, how to do things? Why aren't we aware of our life choices? I am becoming more aware, but I need more guidance and support in how to use the tools. If only we, as women, could be happier doing what we like to do, knowing how to do it well. Who are we depending on for our happiness? I feel that I need to come to understand myself first. I've been to a number of women's groups over the years, and we're not taught to do that. I need to make a choice, have a commitment and work toward it.

I'm in the midst of challenges – the daycare is in a fight with the city to maintain its licence, my marriage is an ongoing battle, we're struggling to keep up with payments for the house and make ends meet. But as I continue to do the Light something must be starting to show. People are making comments such as, "Have you lost weight?" "You look lighter!" "My, you're bright today." Through my inner work and practices I am beginning to catch a glimpse in my heart that my life has meaning.

Spring 1978

Dreams are starting to change me on the inside – knowing they are there and having a way to interpret them. They are so diamond-like. They show me so many different facets of myself – different personality aspects and roles. They help me make choices and question whether the way I am acting is the way I really want to be.

I return to the Ashram at the beginning of June for a dream workshop. A character named "Lady Able" shows up in my dream and I am encouraged to dialogue with her. Who is this able lady, this capable aspect of myself?

Lady Able tells me she comes from the greenness of the trees, the bushes, grass, moss, and has a pleasant, peaceful life growing with positive ideas. She comes from softness and layering growth of all the textures and colours of the seasons, and is not one to sit still. She is always growing and doing things, but her energy is directed and powerful.

I admit that I am afraid of change. She encourages me to consider the subtle changes from trees in bud to leafing, the surprising change of green flower bud to an open flower.

"Become aware of the subtle changes, work to make the seed grow. Water it, care for it, let the sunshine glow on it. Use it when it is ready. Once you know life force will only be positive, you will not be afraid of change.

"Allow yourself to look at all parts – open and exposed, darkness and light. You want to experience to the fullest. Realize you are a changing flowing entity. You may be one way one day and another the next. Make use of it. Be daring and not closed or predictable."

I ask, "What about the people who know me? What will they think?"

"Tell them you have not *become*, yet. You are working on yourself to find all your nooks and crannies. Must you be static and steady? Even a rock changes! Show all of your parts and express how things are for you."

Lady Able is a voice that has beautiful things to say. She speaks poetry and ancient wisdom and I am overcome with joy at discovering her. After this dialogue a hummingbird comes to my window and just hovers there, looking at me.

It seems quite magical, as though I've received a gift that shouldn't be denied or pushed away.

Summer 1978

I listen to that inner voice and start to look into the darkness as well as the light. I know I have a dark side and I am more aware of it now that I have started working on myself. A few months ago I asked for the darkness because I felt I could handle it all at once. In my dream a bird swooped down into a pond and picked up some black fungus and dropped it onto my head and back. It actually stung me and I literally leaped out of bed. Obviously I couldn't handle it as well as I thought. Later in the week I dreamed of being in a delicatessen where there was the same black stuff, but cut into slices. The message – take it in smaller pieces.

I go back to the Ashram for a course based on Swami Radha's brand-new Kundalini book[1]. There is a lot of celebration around the publication of this book, and I am able to buy a signed copy. The class is led by two ashram residents, Swami Radha's students. In one of the reflections on the first *cakra*, they ask us to investigate sex and marriage. I need to bring awareness into what is a dark area for me.

After the birth of my second child I realized that I had only so much energy and that two children and a husband making demands on me were too much. I couldn't cope and went into a black time. Coupled with this was the myth that women could and should be able to cope. I was not and I had no desire to do so. I became uninterested in sex. And there was the myth that women over thirty-five were supposed to experience their most fulfilling years sexually.

---

1 Swami Sivananda Radha, *Kundalini Yoga for the West* (Kootenay Bay, BC: Timeless Books, 2004). The book was first released in 1978.

And here I was not at all interested. I wondered if I was in some way misdirected or abnormal. But our relationship in other terms was not all that damaged. We still had the same commitment to each other and the sense of responsibility to the children.

Maybe people can go through stages, and celibacy is one stage. This is a new idea. Can I look at our marriage in a positive instead of negative light? What if this phase is a progression and not a breakdown? Then I can see a direction and purpose for our marriage and I can change my guilt, confusion and worry into looking at the good aspects. I think this clarification will revitalize my love. My husband is a choice as a friend and we have made certain choices together. And so far, the basic feeling of love is still there, even through conflicts.

Tonight when I repeat the Divine Light Invocation I remember back to my first satsang at the Ashram. Because I couldn't explain it, I kept the experience hidden, even from myself. It felt as though a Divine Light walked right up and into my heart centre and plastered herself right into me – Light and warm – and everything glowed and radiated out of me. I know the Light is there if I peel away the layers. And if I have it, everyone has it. It's just a matter of realization.

I realize the more I come to the Ashram, the more I have a real desire to make a spiritual commitment. I'm questioning myself and my use of speech. I want to watch my energy levels. Where does my energy go?

Winter 1978–79

Looking over the events since the summer and my intent to use my energies with more awareness, I see great gaps and very hard conflicts. Dreams have kept me going.

They give me a new perspective that seems wiser than my conscious mind.

In the darkest time I went to a Hatha Yoga workshop in Calgary, and it renewed me enough to get over the emotional hurdle. When I do a posture the energy doesn't stop at my fingertips or skin. There is no body-mind split. All is one. It has given me confidence in my body and in myself.

At the daycare centre we had very difficult times but miraculously things are working out. I am really fond of the evolving structure of the centre, the freedom to explore my teaching techniques, the people I work with, the children, but it doesn't give me much time or money to get to the Ashram or to support my family, which I am doing on my own now. I wonder if I should look for a better paying job?

Arthur's unemployment insurance ran out, which used to give us just the edge we needed. Now he feels he isn't contributing and has collapsed in many ways. He is not completely happy being at home and I am reacting to his drinking, smoking, sleeping and lack of direction. I am angry and scared that a pattern is developing of him being sick, doing nothing, drinking, depression. I don't know how to deal with it. I recently discovered he has been taking money and that our accounts are overdrawn. I have no experience managing money. How little can we live on?

When I found out Susan and Russell were going to the three-month Yoga Development Course at the Ashram this January, at first I was envious. But then I had a dream of large, lush, healthy plants growing in their garden, and I felt supportive and joyful for them after that.

Two dreams with Swami Radha encourage me to deepen my connection. In October I had a dream message, "Meditate with the moon." Swami Radha holds my head and mothers me. In December I dream that Swami Radha tells me I should come back home to the Ashram as I am not doing enough spiritual work. I say I am baking bread and writing in my diary.

Today I chant with Josephine and her friend, who has just been diagnosed with a brain tumour, then visit Sara and her newly adopted baby. Arthur says our accounts are overdrawn; money is a problem. I bake with Clea and create an affirmation for myself, "I am secure and I am doing the right thing."

My New Year's impressions are of great darkness. Susan has gone to the YDC, Arthur is lacking initiative, the daycare is in a muddle, I am overworked. I want to be perfect – giving, loving, open, understanding, concerned. How do I feel when I make a mistake and speak unkindly or become envious or ignore someone? I feel badly and the consequences are so great. Garth and Clea pick up the words and attitudes and Arthur is not helped by my unkindness.

I want to be a good friend and a fine example, not to be pulled in by others' emotions, but to think clearly. I want to spend time doing yoga each day, to be understanding, to have more time and money for spiritual practice, and to have my family safely looked after.

I read about humility and gratitude in the Kundalini book. Swami Radha says to look for the positive and recount what I have to be grateful for. I am grateful for Clea and her gift of make-believe, for Garth and his health and friendship with Michael, for Arthur and his new determination to find work.

Spring 1979

For the first time our whole family is going to the Ashram. Arthur and I are both nervous as we approach, but it all works out. Our room has a splendid view and it's wonderful to see Susan and Russell, who have stayed on after their YDC teacher training. I have time for my own practices and we connect with the children and with different people who live here. It's Easter and the children love the Easter egg hunt and the hike to Easter Rock, where we all sing uplifting songs into the blue sky. Early one morning while the others are sleeping, Clea and I walk to the beach, play by the water, and I sing "Most Beautiful Mother" as she looks for green rocks. We stop for a few magic moments in the Prayer Room.

When we're back home Garth says he wishes he could live at the Ashram or that we had never gone so he wouldn't know he wanted to live there. Clea asks me about the song we sang and I teach her "Most Beautiful Mother." I overhear Arthur telling friends that the Ashram people have a special look about them. He says it was a lovely "sermon on the mount" for Easter. I am amazed that he is so positive about his experience.

At work, the director's mother dies and she leaves for England. I take over and handle the situation calmly and responsibly. Clea has the measles. University students observe at the daycare and are impressed. Arthur makes dinner – he is drunk and tired. We have a rushed staff meeting, a successful parent meeting, an enlivening yoga class.

In May I return to the Ashram to do the Ten Days of Yoga program, the one that inspired Susan so much.

Everything seems to be here just for me – blossoms, spring flowers, blue clouds of forget-me-nots. It is just so sweet, like heaven. Doing all the practices opens me up to their power and to the beauty of this place. I like the people at the Ashram and how they are living their lives, and I want to be like them.

After chanting the whole world and my body seem to be singing the mantra. I leave the Prayer Room and meet a white butterfly. She does a dance around me. I stop and watch as she dances and dances around. I think she might lead me, but she turns and flits quickly to the sky, landing on a blossom tree and looking like a blossom.

What is the purpose of my life? Last night I had a dream that was almost like an advertisement. I was in a room with two children and they were noisy and disruptive. Then I took them by the hand and together we walked quietly toward the sun. Walking toward the Light is the purpose of my life.

After the Ten Days I'm happy to come home and see everyone. I can look at things differently. It seems easy to do the Divine Light Invocation. Some of my friends are cautious around me; others are curious.

I am overjoyed when Susan and Russell come back to Lethbridge, and we celebrate with a feast. I'm so grateful that they are here with their new skills and yoga teacher training. Their presence reassures me. I appreciate their directness, straightness and industry, and I have the spiritual support I have so desperately been missing. I want others to recognize the Light in them so they will see it in themselves. But my friends and husband don't seem to want to see positive change; they are trained to look for the negative. It's almost as if they aren't really looking or listening but only thinking what they always think. I must be strong enough to follow my own path, whether or not others approve.

Daily life goes on. I go shopping, buy material for living room curtains, make carob cookies, visit with a friend, swim with Clea, argue with Arthur, make Clea's dress, chant. Garth talks about immortality and which part of him could last forever. I read him *The Cat Who Went to Heaven*[2]. The next day I have a good discussion with Arthur about his work around the house and talk to the kids about the Light. Garth is interested in yoga poses so we do some together. Visit with Susan. A friend has a nervous breakdown and I support her in the Light.

I have a dream that we are in a house waiting for the end to come. We are in a foreign city. There is a group of us. We can see the city laid out. It is an Eastern city. Everyone prepares by getting books, putting on jewelry, writing things down. This vortex of energy and Light turns everything to brilliance and it disappears.

Summer 1979

I make a quick weekend trip to the Ashram with the children. I'm doing the Straight Walk workshop and they are in the Children's Program. We walk down to Main House and see Swami Radha, who is very friendly. She looks at me intently, as though she is seeing me in a way that I can't see myself. She says, "Oh, so you've come back." There is something in her voice – as if she is not just talking about me coming back to the Ashram for another visit, but about me coming back from another time. I feel close to her. What does she know?

The instructions for the Straight Walk are to walk between two points, gather facts, observe how I walk, experiment, watch my thoughts, write it all down. I find myself frightened and tense at first, then wobbly and unsteady. I have trouble turning around and try walking sideways so I won't have to change directions. I tiptoe for a while. As I continue walking I relax and feel my feet firmly on

---

2   Elizabeth Coatsworth and Lynd Ward, *The Cat Who Went To Heaven* (New York: Aladdin Paperbacks, 1990).

the floor. The window provides perspective and fresh air. In the other direction I walk to an imaginary line. When I turn swiftly my children suddenly appear at the window watching me, and I wave for them to go upstairs to our room. When I start thinking about them sadness comes over my body. I step across the imaginary line to write my paper.

It is my relationship with Arthur that is on my mind. I'm afraid to face the facts and take action to turn things around. Our relationship is shaky and I've been tiptoeing around it or sidling away, unable to change directions. I feel now that if there is any relationship I want with him it would be as a friend – not easy because of his negativity, but possible because of what we have been through for fourteen years. As a friend I would have to tell him how I feel about him, what I am doing, and what I expect. Money would have to be accounted for, work described, room allotted, separation allowed.

I leave the Ashram with two sleeping children and hugs from the instructor and drive home by moonlight. I am mulling over my life as I drive, remembering back to how I met Arthur. It was October 1963 when two friends and I were in a serious car accident near Hope, BC. I was driving and blinded by car lights coming straight at me. We went over "Honeymoon Corner," a 500-foot embankment that no one had ever survived. We came out with just a few injuries and our story made front-page news. I learned later that Arthur knew one of my friends in the car, and he read about us on the lit-up news signboard outside the Hotel Vancouver.

I met him a year later and was blinded by his blazing intellect and his reputation in the arts and music. He was bisexual, and I was attracted to his gentleness and kindness, and he loved to be with me. I liked his way of talking and including women, his being the centre of attention in a fascinating group of avant garde friends, and his orderliness.

He was also the furthest thing I could imagine from my truck-driving father.

We married the following year. I continued teaching while he went back to university as a mature student, politically active and writing reviews for the newspaper. But we grew apart, especially after the birth of the children. Now we keep heading in different directions. I am on this path of Light and he is drinking, depressed and unemployed.

We arrive home from the Ashram at 2:30 a.m. The next day I tell Susan that the children and I traveled 500 miles to the Ashram and back on the weekend so I could talk about Arthur and myself. She said it would have been surprising if I hadn't talked about the relationship. Maybe I needed the distance.

I know I have to address this issue of our marriage and take some kind of action. I build up my courage and ask Arthur if we can meet. After the children are in bed we sit together for an in-depth talk. I bring up my concerns and tell him about my sense of direction. He seems receptive and agrees that we should have separate rooms. I will move upstairs to the third floor, where I can have my own bedroom plus a prayer room and he will stay on the second floor. He also tells me he is very interested in helping to build the Temple of Light at the Ashram. The Temple has been a long-time dream of Swami Radha's. A foundation was built more than ten years ago, but she says there needs to be harmony at the Ashram before the Temple will manifest. I feel touched that Arthur wants to be part of it. And it's so amazing to feel we are finally working together. I am truly excited!

Throughout the week Arthur seems much more at ease and not so negative. I tell him I'm making plans to attend more ashram courses this summer. He supports it and says that it is money well spent.

I return to the Ashram for a course on relaxation and breathing, and then Six Senses in Seven Days, which really pulls the rug out from under me. As I explore my senses and listen to others' observations I am shocked to realize that everything is perception. How can any two people ever communicate with each other when each of us perceives the world so differently?

After the course Arthur comes out and we drive to Princeton with the kids to visit my family. Mom and I talk about purpose. Dad asks if I can cross my legs and stare at my navel yet. On Sunday morning he makes special pancakes for Garth and Clea, then takes them out to pick raspberries. My younger sister Julie helps the kids make a parade with flower garlands around their necks and even around her puppy, Sage, whom the kids adore. Julie has a yoga practice too, and wants to know more about the Ashram. She seems at loose ends after a relationship breakup, so I invite her to Lethbridge in the fall. The kids love her and she's agreed to babysit while Arthur and I take Swami Radha's Life Seals workshop in September.

When we get back home to Lethbridge I start to do a regular mantra practice. I used to chant quietly so I wouldn't disturb Arthur. But now I'm singing out loud and I am consciously working to control my mind. I'm also speaking up. Arthur has changed his views about the Ashram. Maybe he feels threatened, but he has become sharply critical and says he's not in favour of single-pointed discipline. He admits that he has no discipline at all and doesn't apply himself. He says he believes only in the rational mind. How can he cut off a whole part of his mind? How can we work out our differences?

Fall 1979

Tonight is the first time we have satsang in my third-floor prayer room. I feel nervous and exalted about it. I'm also a bit worried about Julie coming this week. And then – in just a few short weeks – Swami Radha will be here to lead a Life Seals workshop at Susan and Russell's house! We've asked all our friends to sign up and have a large group of participants.

When I wake up the moon is at my window, a slim thing. It makes my day beautiful.

Julie arrives and it's a relief somehow to have her here. The kids are excited to see her and Sage. She volunteers at the daycare for a few days and works out so well that she is offered a job.

A nervous day. Swami Radha is here in Lethbridge! In the evening we gather and meet her and start our Life Seals drawings – twenty-seven of them representing different aspects of ourselves, including our essence, mind, senses, strengths and weaknesses, likes and dislikes. We cut out the individual seals and arrange them on a larger sheet so we each have our unique charts. We are all nervous and new to the process.

I volunteer to go first. As we go through the seals and I comment on them I am encouraged to think deeper from my personal experience. It is exciting and daunting at the same time. I see my tendency to please or to try to find the right answer, but the point is to explore the questions and find out what choices I am making, to find out about my mind and how to make it more flexible. Be inquisitive. How does this relate to my life? The teaching style is so potent and so personal.

At one point I look up and observe that I have put all of my pictures in boxes. Protection and limitation. Here I am in front of all my friends not being open. Do I want to feel safe? Am I afraid? What do I think will happen? I think I will disappear, that something I have just recently discovered will be destroyed. I'm not sure if I am strong enough yet to open up. I cannot expose Arthur and myself by letting everyone know what is happening in our marriage. Am I pretending to be someone I am not? Am I afraid people will discover this? Do they know anyway? Do I feel I have to measure up for someone else's benefit?

In the silence I feel Swami Radha is holding me in the Light. Although I don't speak I feel understood and not pressured. There is time to speak and time to listen.

Listening to other people I can see how universal these human problems are. If I hold someone in an image, as I have with Arthur, it becomes harder to take responsibility for what is really happening. We are pretending it is working and it's not. Why can't I talk about it? If I can't accept the truth, why do I think it's easier to accept a lie?

This process of clarification does not promise happiness but it does offer direction, self-knowledge and change. Just what I need. It is an exciting, enlightening weekend.

On Sunday evening we gather for satsang and Swami Radha describes her first satsangs in India. She encourages us to meet together and inspire each other. She passes a candle around so we can each offer a prayer to the person next to us. I pass the candle to Arthur with a prayer that he be illuminated by the Light and that his road be bright.

Silence. Swami Radha seems to be breathing in a way that brings peace and expansion to the whole room. As I breathe I am being filled and stretched. I realize growing into Light is a commitment. After satsang I tell Swami Radha I am very thankful for her presence and insights. How can I thank her? She says to do the Divine Light Invocation for her. I am pleased because I have been visualizing her in the Light once a day since I first met her two years ago.

On Thanksgiving I decide that I will start putting her in the Light three times a day for the next year. I write a card to her to express my commitment. As I am sending it I feel my whole body react. How will it be received? Am I doing a strange thing? I send it anyway.

I have a dream that I look at Swami Radha and smile with a feeling of oneness, and I kiss her on the cheek. She says if I kiss her on the cheek, I must always have my feet on the ground.

Today I receive a note back from her. I am completely thrilled. Along with the note, she sent a section proof from her new book, Aphorisms[3]. The section is called "Especially for Women," and it is illustrated with a drawing of a goddess on a crescent moon. One of the aphorisms really speaks to me: "The major problem facing woman is to develop her emotional independence. She can only do this by recognizing her Divine nature."

I feel as though Swami Radha is encouraging me. Her response confirms that she knows me and that her help doesn't stop when the workshop ends. Why would she choose this part of her new book? Her message, coming in this different way, confirms my dream. To accept the Divine I have to know what I am doing. I have to be practical, to be here with my feet on the ground. I need to develop emotional independence.

I get the message but my marriage continues to be rough. Arthur applies for jobs and doesn't get them, then becomes more depressed. It culminates in an accident he has with both children in the car. The front of the van is bashed in but no one is hurt. I am distraught. He is in despair.

---

3   Swami Radha's book, Aphorisms, is now out of print.

The Path of Liberation

Winter 1980

I've heard that doing the Divine Light Invocation ten times a day for forty days brings a miracle. I'm trying it... also to prepare for the mind workshop with Swami Radha coming up in Calgary this spring.

In my day to day, I have tea and talk with my women friends, do yoga, go to group, go to work – working things out with the director, the staff, the parents. I cook and bake bread. People I know die and others get sick.

In our weekly Kundalini class we're exploring the first *cakra* – sex, love, birth, death and the sense of smell. Julie has joined the group, too, and the children like smelling everything with us. Clea says my third-floor prayer room smells like the Ashram.

I have a dream that blueberries are growing very fat and juicy by a stream.

Spring 1980

In the mind workshop in Calgary, Swami Radha challenges us

to clarify how our minds have created our lives. I see how my mind creates patterns and then gets caught in them. How does that work in my marriage, my career and my spiritual life?

Why did I marry? My mind was ready to accept the familiar cultural pattern that I should marry. I was a product of the 1950s when a woman was thought to need a man to be complete. I married someone I felt was kind and understanding as well as stimulating artistically and intellectually, and I married to have children, to be supported and to be happy. I didn't challenge this concept and now I'm turning it upside down. But in doing so, I am exploring new areas and becoming more aware. However, seeing other couples separate and remarry similar people, I would rather work on this one marriage with a feeling of commitment than repeat the same pattern. Plus I want to avoid the added sorrow to the children. With my husband, I try not to assume too much. I go out to work and he stays home to look after the house and children. Every day is an opportunity to watch my reactions to him and to work on the relationship.

What is my work pattern? I have a very fulfilling job that provides a service. I have dedicated a lot of time and energy to establishing the daycare centre and now teaching in it. I creatively choose projects and experiences that are challenging for the level the children are at, being encouraging yet demanding of what they can do. But just recently my mind was jogged by another job possibility and I started to look at options. I am coming to terms with service, self-worth, professionalism and money. I see that I must look more closely at my work and re-evaluate my interests, outlook and attitude.

With spirituality I've had an underlying concept that being spiritual means setting myself apart like a nun or a minister. It is a relatively new thought that I can live my spiritual life as I am. In the newness my mind makes the practices special. But as I do the practices I realize I must take them out of the mind and into my daily events and relationships. As I see the useful changes in my body and mind I become more aware of what I do with my energy. I want to learn from both my marriage and my job not to be complacent and not to put too many expectations onto my spiritual life. I am involved in yoga groups where I gather with others to stimulate and refresh the direction I want my mind to be going. We come together for Kundalini and dream groups as well as satsang, where community is shared in a very meaningful way. At the end of the day I write about how I have handled my attitudes and what changes I am making.

My life is vastly different from what it was two years ago, and the reason is the clarity I've gained from the teachings. I am just starting to unlock the limitations of my mind, and I am open to opportunities within the limitations.

At the end of the workshop Swami Radha hugs me in a warm, loving embrace. I am thrilled and grateful to be so close to her, to understand the depths of her compassion and to see the changes in my life. This is my miracle. Driving back to Lethbridge, Susan, Julie and I are in a good space – thrilled and grateful.

Our whole family goes to the Ashram for Easter again this year. I type out the paper on what I learned from the mind workshop, and when I give a copy to Swami Radha she asks me to bring my family over for lunch the next day. I am so excited! We eat lunch with her at her home, Many Mansions, and I don't feel nervous. It is very pleasant, but why am I here with this family? She treats us as guests. We don't know what to say. The children don't speak up. Arthur seems dazed. We talk about weather and work. She gives many suggestions.

When we get back to Lethbridge my life keeps expanding. I am asked to be on a panel to speak about daycare at a conference – ten whole minutes. I'm not used to being the centre of attention and speaking in front of a large group. I'm worried and spend a lot of time preparing but when the moment comes I find it easy and exciting to do. People listen and I discover I actually have something to say from all my years of teaching and setting up the daycare. I have conviction about my methods of trusting children's intelligence and giving them creative learning centres within a structured environment. I can see I am gaining knowledge through experience and I feel good about it. I wouldn't have been able to do this a few years ago. Part of the confidence comes from preparing papers and speaking in Kundalini class.

I want to take lots of courses at the Ashram this summer. I write to the daycare board requesting school holidays in lieu of a salary increase, which I know they can't afford. They respond affirmatively and I happily sign up for as many ashram courses as I can. Julie is just back from the Ten Days of Yoga course, looking good. She appears to be really finding out what she wants.

Mom phones that Dad has been having trouble with his heart. He is having more tests and has bypass surgery scheduled so he can be more active again.

Summer 1980

Our marriage is shaky, almost dying. Can it be revived? It feels like a miracle when Arthur agrees to come to the Ashram with me for a Couples Life Seals workshop. There are other couples and it is somehow reassuring hearing that they have almost the same problem as ours – not being able to communicate.

In the Life Seals there is something you see. Up to that point you haven't seen it, then you see it. With Arthur's Life Seals I see both sides – the smoke that covers everything, a smokescreen that hides the facts; and a little plant with a flower and a fence around it, protecting this tender part that might grow if given a chance.

We've both drawn our house to represent family. His house is small and surrounded in a dusty tornado while mine is large, gorgeous and central. He says he's happy at home, but it doesn't show. The van, which he says symbolizes a way out and freedom to move, is obviously much more appealing for him.

Something is there but it is out of proportion.

As we work through our separate Life Seals and then look at them together, I feel my commitment to the marriage is strong, but I'm becoming impatient. I have my own direction and am concerned with his lack of initiative.

Will it work? I hear different ways that other couples have been dealing with their relationships. I have hope and confidence that when we get back something will change. The man I married fifteen years ago is my husband who I said I would love and care for, and I still think I should.

We have a beginning spark.

Just back from the workshop and I am alone in the house. The phone rings and it is my sister Bonnie calling to say that Dad has died. I can't believe it! We would have visited him in two weeks. Try to think. A muddle. Where is he now? I am alone, looking at the clouds, thinking maybe he is up there. But how would I see him? It's just me, the wind and the clouds.

Julie and I fly out to Princeton with the children. The ceremony is excellent. Mom feels much calmer afterward. It is a Masonic service and they do a ceremony similar to the Divine Light, then each of them puts a sprig of evergreen on the coffin. We add our flowers – Mom, a white rose; me, a marigold. Later we go back to the grave. It looks lovely covered with flowers.

I realize it was just a week ago that Arthur and I did the Life Seals workshop, and I had many thoughts about death. Also our Kundalini group is reflecting on death. The day after the Life Seals my father died. It is as if the images of death and dying were projected for me to see, helping to unblock the passages of my mind by giving an indication of what was in store.

As I work on clarifying my life I am becoming more aware of these underlying connections and see the guidance that is there. It allows for strange occurrences. After the funeral I am alone in my room and see an angel above me – close and feathery, glowing, very white. It is almost like a cloak descending or a helper showing me there is another realm. Children often tell me that they've seen angels and they like to draw them. I, too, have seen an angel and have accepted it and added it to the forms in my world.

My sister Bonnie wanted some kind of message that Dad was all right, and I suggested that she look and listen very carefully. Driving home the next day she saw lightning flash over her house in a cloudless sky. She was thrilled by the communication. It requires a leap of faith to move out of the solid world.

Coming back home to Lethbridge I'm disappointed to find the house a mess and the smell of smoke everywhere. While we were gone Arthur's cigarette started a fire on one of the old armchairs. Although he's removed the burnt-up chair, the smell remains.

The Path of Liberation workshop at the Ashram is supposed to be for advanced students, but I am so eager to learn from Swami Radha that my application has been accepted.

The first assignment Swami Radha gives us is to brainstorm mind and consciousness. I start out enthusiastically – anything on the mind that comes to mind. And immediately I am caught in my structure. How far can I stretch the space that is contained in this body? What is the constraint that keeps the whole thing from exploding? I think of the Light and how it permeates the container, opening it to knowledge. I direct and surrender so every level of consciousness is filled. By saying that, I am confirming that there *are* different levels to be opened and filled.

Tonight there is a full moon lighting the path as I walk up from the Prayer Room. Walking a path of light and taking a course called the Path of Liberation. It seems the whole world is a mandala, laid out for a purpose – to show me that I am receiving energy from one endless source.

Swami Radha asks us to write about the symbols and the mantras of the first three *cakras*. Although I've studied her Kundalini book and answered some of the questions, I haven't concentrated on the images and mantras before. The *cakras* look complex, with many-headed gods and goddesses and fierce weapons; the mantras seem esoteric, sprinkled with Sanskrit. I decide to follow what Swami Radha's guru, Swami Sivananda, did to clear the air and his mind – chant *Om* loudly three times. Then I will write. I am willing or desperate enough to allow a process that seems to depend on some other dimension, just letting whatever is there come through.

Sitting outside overlooking the lake, I start the practice. As I do my first *Om* I hear a humming sound. I stop. A hummingbird is hovering right beside me looking, attentive, pausing. A few years ago a hummingbird outside my window was a messenger confirming my creativity following my dialogue with Lady Able. Now this hummingbird is even closer – no barriers. Is it hurt? Why does it stay so long? Suddenly its wings are in action – fibrous, luminous, whirling, straight ahead. What a start!

When I relax and trust this other level something else seems to come through – the messengers and the message. The next day I hear that many of the experienced students had stayed up all night struggling to piece together their understanding of the Kundalini system with their lives. My reflections are more like poetry. After I read them there is silence. The next evening we reflect on the next three *cakras* and mantras, and again a flow of intuition.

As the workshop progresses I write down the strong feelings that are surfacing…

I feel liberated!

Singing body wants to explode with joy and Light. Do not contain me in your wife and mother role! I am here to do Divine work! I am your container for the Light. Why squeeze and pain me?

Crying, the rain runs out of my eyes. See the world in different ways and radiate instead of drawing in. The water flows from springs inside knowing there is a never-ending source. It flows through outer curves and touches my skin. I have an outer and an inner and they want to meet.

Patterns impressed upon my body, locks that need opening and flexibility. My life, a spiritual reality. Getting in touch with wisdom flowing from the Divine Source, never ending. In that I put my trust…

At the end of the workshop Swami Radha asks me if I like Kundalini, and I say that I do. She asks if I found it strange or strenuous? I say no, and I thank her. I review my notes, sifting through ideas, feeling uplifted and making connections.

Fall 1980

A night of awakening moonlight. At home in my room on
the third storey, I see the big old cottonwood tree glowing
outside and I get up from bed and do a Divine Light. A moth
flutters over me. A dream lingers. I write a poem for Swami
Radha, then do 108 Divine Mother prayers. I hear Arthur
coughing in his room. When we were away at the Ashram a
friend said he seemed immobilized.

In the morning I receive a call from one of his associates
asking about money that Arthur owes him. I am extremely
angry that he hasn't mentioned it. More bills come in that I
hadn't known about. I feel really betrayed and go to the bank
and transfer the money to another account. I tell him and he
looks ashen. What he owes he should pay back. I feel drained.

He is often drinking, in a stupor, or frantic – it's the
source of many of our arguments. Often I hear him drive off
into the night, coming back in the early morning. He has
another life.

October days, hot and windy. I sit in the sun and pull
out dead plants from the garden. Susan is worried about me.
She says I look unhappy. The children at the centre are edgy;
Arthur is extremely miserable.

I'm up early and go to the Sally Ann, then food
shopping, take the kids to a puppet show at the library, clean
the house, bathe Clea, go to the movie set where Garth and
Arthur are working as extras. Garth makes $165 for his part
and opens his own bank account. He gives $5 to Clea. We're
making masks as part of our Kundalini group and Clea, too,
wants to make a mask. I get Arthur a job as the handyman at
the daycare.

In November, on his fiftieth birthday, Arthur is in a foul
mood, afraid of getting old. I try to encourage him to talk.
He doesn't know why he is depressed.

The bank phones that there is one dollar in the account. We go over the books and he admits he applied for a credit card and says he used it to buy more than $400 worth of gas this summer without mentioning it.

Winter 1981

I'm at the end of my rope. The only thing I can think of to do is put Arthur and our marriage in the Light ten times a day. I start in the New Year. On February 4th, my birthday cake is ablaze with forty candles and I feel sad. Where is this life going?

I come home from work one night to find the dog howling and Arthur screaming and falling to the kitchen floor. The honey he was boiling for granola has spilled all over his arm and hand. He is badly burned. He puts his arm under the tap. I try to get him to go with me to the hospital but he refuses. He says he can take care of it himself. I can only stand, helpless. His drinking makes him act like a sleepwalker.

A few days later a terrifying start to the day. I open the door to a man who has papers to repossess our house. Foreclosure. I am hysterical. Arthur admits he has only made two payments in the last five months. He wants to self-destruct. He agrees to go for counseling. I phone Susan and go to the coulees and scream. I phone the Ashram and put us on the prayer list, then phone a lawyer. We can pay in instalments. I can borrow money from Dad's estate.

My body is full of pain. I feel I am holding someone else's garbage on my back. Both children are disturbed and worried about him. How to cope with the kids? Clea has no friends and Garth is putting on weight and having trouble communicating. Garth asks why we fight and I try to tell him how I feel. He thinks Arthur is a good dad.

Arthur has made a plan to go for counseling. It is strange. I feel more compassion for him now. I can hear him better.

Spring 1981

Another windy day in Lethbridge. I walk to the gas company and discover that the bill has been run up and not paid for months. It feels like the last straw. The wind is screaming, howling, sweeping clean. As I walk down the street the wind whips away the bill and the remnants of my marriage. In my mind it is over.

Maybe I expected the Light to heal in a kinder way. I have to accept that what the Light has revealed is what I need to see. This is the miracle.

I re-register the car in my name, have time to buy chocolate eggs and bunnies, and the children and I are off to the Ashram for Easter.

It is quiet here. Garth goes with Robert, one of his favourite residents, on his motorbike and Clea plays with two other girls. Later I talk to Robert. He feels I have been more than accommodating with Arthur and he suggests I make a list of what I expect, have Arthur sign and keep to it. If he stays in the house, he can be a boarder.

I decide to take the Six Week Program this summer. It combines courses with work. Bringing the kids here will be a transition for them and for me. In the back of my mind is a desire to live at the Ashram for two years while Swami Radha is still alive.

When I return home Arthur and I talk at lunch. He agrees to the contract and conditions. I see him as a person with problems that are not something I can solve. I have had expectations that he would change but now I see I have to change my expectations. The ending. How to end? Today the house picture falls off my Life Seals drawing that hangs on the wall.

My day: I take Clea to ballet and make a concerted effort to support Garth. Arthur and I write papers on our marriage – a difficult meeting, feeling I am too close to ask questions. I interpret my dreams, update résumé, see that we have five dollars left in our bank account. I wash all the kitchen walls, dig up the whole garden – stay active, be physical, work off the anxiety.

Early June and Swami Radha is coming back to Lethbridge for a workshop. She arrives at Susan's and I go over and have tea with her. She looks intently at me and asks, "How long has your marriage been crummy? What is he doing?"

At the Mountain pose workshop with Swami Radha, I look at my life and marriage clearly. Standing up for myself. Standing firm. Using *tadasana*, the Mountain pose, in real life. Straightening up and looking squarely at what is in front of me. I can be straight. I can be firm. I am a mountain.

I remember the Straight Walk where I saw that I am wobbly in my relationship with Arthur. Finding the way rocky, not seeing pitfalls, stumbling over the facts that I want support from someone else, that the base is not firm in our relationship. Hard to look through the trees on the mountain slope. I get caught up in the patterns. Reflection creates the open space where I can catch a glimpse of the top.

Each step brings a new view and the vision takes on a different shape. I see the whole mountain as the challenge. I first heard from Swami Radha that Light was available to those who wanted it and that women must stand on their own two feet. Her challenge was like the white brilliance of the snowy peak. I look at the structure of the mountain. It has a base – solid, firm, balanced. I am bringing a firm base into my life, trusting in the Light, asking for help, seeking possibilities, working through, leaving it to the Light once the work is done, and accepting what comes.

The Path of Liberation happens step by step. I work with the groups, satsang, dreams, reflecting on my day and its insights, practising bringing quality into my life. My plan is to go up the mountain, to do in-depth study on myself at the Ashram, to spiritualize the life I am in now by bringing awareness and acceptance, and clearly seeing where I am and what I am doing. The stillness of the pose helps.

Right now I am straightening out the relationship and it is painful. I get caught up in patterns and regrets, and those are the obstacles. But I receive help from the hills. I am truly grateful.

I take my stand. It is up to Arthur to leave and find a job. I need to accept the opportunity to trust in the Light. He says he wants to leave. He says it in an amusing way, as if it's an adventure. He is continuing to drink. He finally tells the kids that he will be leaving in a few days. We do the Light together. He has no plans. He is excited and afraid. I feel tense over what he is doing, numb through the day.

His first day gone. It's lunchtime and the kids are upset that lunch isn't ready. But then they understand. Garth asks how long Dad will be away. I say until September. Then we will meet again and decide next steps.

It seems as though the way now is a legal separation. Arthur has left but I could never have accepted that this was a helping situation had I not received all the help that was given to me. The Mountain workshop was perfect timing. I got so much support from the group and Swami Radha.

I get dressed up and go to the lawyer. In order to implement the separation process I'll have to find Arthur or go to the RCMP. I call his sister in Halifax and she gives me a number in Vancouver. There is no answer at first, then Arthur comes on. He seems jolly. I feel angry that he assumes no responsibility.

Summer 1981

Entering the Ashram, Swami Radha gives me a big hug. She asks me about the separation and says I have done well, but there is still a heaviness.

In the Six Week Program, the teachers are asking more of me. They say I am clearer and they encourage me to participate more. I am experienced and have something to offer. Why the soft voice? Why does my voice trail off? Sometimes it just doesn't seem worth it to talk. I am trying to get myself out of the mud.

Clea and I walk by the lake and pick wild raspberries. Garth works with the ashram men and enjoys being with them. Swami Radha hugs me and I tell her I love her, does she know? I like working – whether it's shoveling gravel, washing windows in the Prayer Room, doing dishes, folding sheets in the laundry room, or working with the children in the Children's Program. Often Swami Radha asks me to sit beside her at meals. I wonder why.

In class today we are reflecting on a verse from the Gita: "Tell me decisively, what is good for me. I am Thy disciple. Instruct me who has taken refuge in Thee." I go to the Beach Prayer Room, do the Light and chant to Tara. I want to be receptive to the message of this verse. I feel sad and confused as to actions.

The image of Tara appears that I had visualized one evening in satsang. She has her scarves flying and her foot ready to step down. She is quite big and I see myself standing in *tadasana* beside her. She is very beautiful and I ask her to tell me decisively what is good for me.

She picks me up in her arms and rocks me like a baby or a small child. I look just as I look now, the same clothes and feelings. I can see her rocking me and I can feel the movement. She is very gentle. I ask her what actions I should do and she keeps me in her arms. I feel very secure and safe and part of her. I keep asking and she keeps rocking. I kiss her on the cheek and it is very soft and petal-like. I remember Swami Radha's embrace. I realize the challenges will appear. The action is to do what comes my way, knowing I am in her arms.

We celebrate Swami Radha's Silver Jubilee, her twenty-five years of *sanyas*, with many festivities. The children place the garlands they have made around each person, and everyone dedicates a rose to Swami Radha. It brings up beautiful feelings. Julie comes out for the weekend and takes a long time leaving. I give her a hug and wish her well. She's helping to care for the house while we're here and says Arthur is in and out of the house, evasive. She is planning to take the Yoga Development Course in January.

Arthur phones to say he has a university job for six months. He will come to the Ashram for evaluation of our situation in a few weeks. When he arrives I see his fear. In our meeting I try to be honest. We work out details, going slowly until everything clicks and we are both satisfied.

A visit with Swami Radha. She asks my direction and I tell her that I want to take the three-month Yoga

Development Course. I will have enough money. The children love it here and they seem more well adjusted after our time this summer. I give her a special brooch as a sign of my gratitude.

I am in a dance between the Ashram and life.

Fall/Winter 1981

Back in Lethbridge I paint the kitchen chairs orange, pick veggies from the garden, look for a bike for Garth and teach Clea to ride her bike. Susan comes for tea and long talks. I wax the hardwood floors, clean the kitchen cupboards and drawers. I take Garth to a Unicef concert at the Sportsplex where his grade six choir sings of the potential for goodness. It makes me realize why I went into teaching – the love, caring, togetherness, ripeness and richness of their young lives. I talk to Arthur about his plans, what he is doing and how we communicate. It seems very open and directed. He promises to pay for the children.

In December, Swami Radha comes to Lethbridge and offers a workshop on the symbolism of *savasana*, the Death pose. My reflections lift me to the next level…

Riding on a cloud of breath everything becomes harmony and comfort in the surrender to the breath and Light. Where is the tension and resistance now? Where is the fear? In three weeks I will be dying to the world I am in. In three weeks I leave Lethbridge, my house, my friends, my groups, my job, my marriage. I will not physically be here. I will be residing somewhere else. I am going toward a vortex of Light and knowledge, which keeps calling me, intriguing me – the Ashram. My purpose is to bring as much Light and awareness to my life as possible. Cooperating with my path by taking the YDC makes it more possible.

My work for the next three weeks is to prepare and plan what we will physically need for our stay – to make my job as workable as possible for the next person to take it over, to clearly and legally put our separation in order, to burn my resentments and recount the benefits from having served each other in this marriage for sixteen years.

Death may be the hardest posture, but the groundwork has been laid and has only to be acted upon. At the death of my father I found a renewed strength in the teachings of the Light. I could see that the physical body had gone but I could crystallize the strengths he had given me. This experience gives me insight into essence.

I receive the blessings and the teachings of Swami Radha and the teachers of the Ashram with gratitude. It is through seeing how they live their lives that I want to do the same. They give selfless service, help and guide people like me, and are so connected to the Light. Their example sets up a yearning in me and gives me the courage to face myself. The teachings have shown me how precious my body is, how necessary and fascinating my mind, and how my life can become a spiritual life…

The Diamond in the Lotus

Winter 1982

As I walk to the office to pay for the Yoga Development
Course I have an emotional attack. I can't do this! How can
I look after the children and be involved in such an intensive
three-month program? How can I drive them up that steep,
snowy, slippery hill to school every morning, especially when
I'm supposed to be in class? What about the children – won't
they feel lonely and alienated going to a new school? Should
I really be here? I sadly express my concerns to Eleanor in the
office. She is sympathetic but encourages me to keep going.
Other participants arrive and I have a sinking feeling that I'm
out of my league. I try to keep an open mind and suspend
judgement. Julie is here for the course too, and she helps us
arrange the room. It's homey.

The first day of school and the children are thrilled with
it and love sleigh-riding down the hill afterward.

The evening before the YDC starts Swami Radha invites
me to Many Mansions. I come in from the dark blackness
outside and she greets me and leads me to the Sun Room, her
private sitting room and office. It's the first time I've been in
here and it is filled with light and warmth. She welcomes me

back, asks about the children, and then sits, twisting a Rubik's Cube. She starts thinking out loud of ways I could stay on at the Ashram. She says she has always known I would be here.

I want to be close to her. I want to be open and confident enough to be her disciple, to bring her whatever I have, whatever I am. I don't want to stay in the outer circle. I want to come into this place of Light. I build up my courage and ask, "May I call you Mataji?"

"Do you know what it means?"

"Mother," I respond.

"Inviting that intimacy means I can meddle in your life. Are you ready for that?" she asks.

"I am."

I feel enveloped in her love as I return to my room. "Mataji!"

The next day I receive a scholarship for the course from the Alberta Heritage Fund. A confirmation! When I tell the kids Garth asks, "Does that mean we can stay longer?" I feel on top of the world.

This morning the yoga class runs late. I leave at my usual time before end relaxation to drive the kids to school. Two tries up the unploughed road. The first time we slide off at the corner, push the car out of the snowbank and try again, successfully.

Breakfast, then back to class. Today is Guided Imagery, one of the first intensive workshops of the program. The instructor leads us in visualizing a house, exploring it, and finding something precious. My experience feels real and overpowering, like a gift.

In the visualization I come up the walk to Swami Radha's house and face the orange door. Should I knock or just enter? I pause before opening, then step into what feels like a sacred space. The walls of the first room are lined with books. The other rooms have sunshine streaming in and beautiful altars with images of Divine Mother. I find a secret door that opens to outside and stroll through the garden to the lotus pond. I am drawn to an open white lotus. Looking inside to the centre, I see a brilliant diamond shimmering with Light.

A diamond in the lotus – I know it is for me.

It is almost tangible as I open my eyes.

Inspiring moments of the day. Cold biting my legs, stillness of snow on the trees, the road bare and easy to drive, singing "Rejoice" with the kids on the way to school, hot porridge and brown sugar, icicles hanging from windows, Swami Radha wearing dark blue sapphires, holding the children, chanting to Divine Mother.

My life has transformed. I am not hiding or protecting myself anymore and I've created a clear pathway from a foundation of devotion, work and reflection up to my innermost self, my essence. My latest Life Seals show me this. Right at the centre I've drawn an orange. Orange – the colour of renunciation. All the swamis here wear orange. I see renunciation as a process of letting go of preconceived ideas. In the back of my mind is the desire to dedicate my basic nature and my path to the Most High.

The orange is an offering at the feet of Tara, the Divine Mother of compassion. Tara is a great help and I can talk to her easily. I ask her to show me the path that my renunciation might take. I offer myself up as a servant to the Most High. I can visualize Tara clearly. I have faith that I can handle whatever she presents me. It may not be the way I have always done it and I may have to give up some of my views of myself, but in doing what is before me my life takes on more meaning and I am receptive to what comes back.

Beside her I've drawn the diamond in the lotus from

the guided visualization last week. The diamond represents clarity and the lotus receptivity; together they create a whole. This seems like a good path to follow, one that demands responsibility and inspiration.

On this day I have a vision of an embroidery of Tara. I make a pact with the Divine: if I receive an embroidered Tara, I will take it as a sign to stay at the Ashram as a resident for two years. I feel restless and fearful of looking squarely at the question of *sanyas*. But it is coming up for me, too, this desire to be a swami.

A marvelous sunny day – February 2nd, the anniversary of Mataji's *sanyas* day. I promise myself to sit with her at lunch if possible, and I do. She talks about selfishness and the Divine law and tells me afterward that she spoke loudly so that the person next to me would get the message. I am thrilled to be in her confidence and to glimpse her methods.

At supper Mataji asks me to join her at the table filled with February birthday celebrants, a group of Aquarians that includes residents and swamis. She asks Clea to hand out different gifts that she has for each of us. When I open my small box, I find a few rice kernels. She tells me they are from her own *sanyas* initiation and I should keep them on my altar. And there is a photograph of Tara, which she had embroidered herself. An embroidered Tara! It's the promised sign of my two-year stay! Such an auspicious day – I feel like I am in seventh heaven!

Straight Walk. I am walking back and forth between the stack of orange chairs and the supply cupboard door in the laundry room at the Guest Lodge. Last year in the Six Week Program I had happy times here, folding fresh sheets, preparing for guests, being of service. The orange chairs symbolize the Ashram, all the workshops when I have sat on these chairs, all the learning that has happened here. Orange again, the colour of renunciation – start with a little, Swami Radha said. She always makes everything practical so it is easy to take the steps. I think of the integrity of the Ashram. It's different from any other place I have ever known – the honesty and straightforward approach. Each time there is so much to learn.

The door has a golden sheen – my life takes on different meaning; things look bright. But brighter also means seeing what I need to work on. Work with Light toward clarity. I have a treasure house, a golden opportunity. Who has the key to the supply cupboard door? Residents. Could I be a resident? Could I be a renunciate?

As I walk back and forth, I move with ease. It is rhythmical now and it feels right. I can move toward renunciation and I know I will do it. It feels good to have made the decision. I come back later at lunch and actually carry an orange chair to my room to make it real for myself. Some day…

The idea of residency at the Ashram is a little frightening to me. Why? The obstacles are my concepts of how I should or shouldn't be. It's not acceptable because I have children. My friends won't understand. I don't have the money. There isn't room at the Ashram. I should further my education. Susan is leaving Lethbridge and we will need another teacher there. I have a house there. Ordinary people don't live at ashrams. It is a secret desire and I shouldn't say it out loud or it will disappear. I'm not sure I could do it.

I want to do it! It would make me happy! The decision is valid but I need to find out more facts.

Swami Radha gives a talk in the evening about making the bridge between the unconscious and conscious. She says that irrational qualities are not only okay, but needed. She is off for six weeks in India to revisit Sivananda Ashram. I am clear that I want to make the two-year commitment. I can see how my fears are often ungrounded.

It's hard to go beyond where I am, but as the course progresses over the three months I gain so much confidence. This morning I am up in the Headstand for the first time – confirmation that I can turn my world upside down! I see my kids watching at the window and I fall out of the pose, laughing.

As we approach spring, the course shifts and I'm up early for my first day of teaching a Hatha Yoga class. It feels very natural and goes well. All day I'm lifted by a surge of spring energy and I run wherever I'm going. I am also excited about doing the thirty book reports, which are required to become a certified teacher. I get a start on them today. Arthur calls to say he misses the kids and is lonely. He plans to come out to see them later in the spring.

A Rose Ceremony marks the end of the course. Clear spring light and oranges for *prasad*. I have discovered so much about myself through the YDC and feel grounded in the Light and ready to renounce. Now I know how to keep my attention focused on the Light as people dive into their process and I dive into mine. It's an invaluable gift.

Spring 1982

I'm catapulted out of the familiar schedule of the YDC and into this new course of working and living at the Ashram until the end of the summer. Mataji returns. There are many new people coming to live here. Will there be room for us? Should we sell the house? I need help to make the changes. I'm losing my nerve…

At supper Mataji talks to another woman interested in residency. I hear her say that only so many people can stay here because of limited accommodation, electricity, and so on. She talks about surrender and how everything doesn't always work out the way we plan. Is the message really for me? Is this her kind way of telling me? The next day I make an appointment to discuss and clarify the possibilities.

Meeting at Many Mansions with Mataji and the senior residents, I look around and see that they are all concerned. I keep listening and keep the Light flowing. I don't need to say much but I appreciate the way they go into all aspects – the pros and cons – so thoroughly. Afterward, a word with Mataji. She says she doesn't know what my Divine Committee has in mind. We have to wait and see.

Arthur calls to say he is coming and the kids are excited and nervous. When he arrives, he takes them to town for shopping. I see he is making an effort, but he looks so unhealthy and forlorn. It makes me feel very sad.

I have another conversation with Swami Radha and she brainstorms numerous ideas for earning money. Then she questions my direction. "What do you think you need?" she asks.

"I need time at the Ashram. I need time to work in this community with the devotional aspect because I feel there is something to learn."

She responds, "That may not have anything to do with learning. Learning can happen anywhere. So what do you think it is? What do you need that the Ashram can give you?"

"I would say it has to do with Divine Mother."

"So you need the devotion, the nourishment, the atmosphere, the conversation. Because the conversations here may go out to worldly affairs but they always come back to the spiritual. And a lot of people have a deep, true sense of gratefulness to be here. Keep looking into possibilities."

I follow through and find out that our house would sell at a price much lower than the money we need. It doesn't look promising.

Mataji is leading our dream group through the summer. Tonight she is fierce in her love and compassion. I think of her greatness – how she worries about all of us, trying to help us, planning for us, accepting us as part of the Divine plan. We all tell ourselves what we need to know.

What is my relationship to Mataji? Sometimes Light comes right through her eyes and I feel it in my heart rushing out. I don't even need to be near her and her Light fills me. There is no time, no in-between. Sometimes I am so grateful that every minute is a whisper of a prayer of gratitude. I look back to the stiffness and darkness I lived in and can hardly recognize myself.

Then I wonder about my sincerity. I have seen others come and go, finding it hard to keep the commitment. Why do I want to be here? Is it enough to want to be near her, to help in whatever way I can? Are there other things I need to do? I search, I plan, I think of everything. I still want to be here, to be near. So I say to Divine Mother that if it isn't possible, make the desire go away or give me the strength to overcome whatever stands in my way.

A great sadness comes over me. I have no money. The house will not sell by September and even if it did, it's not enough. We will have to leave. Nothing is going according to my plan. But the source of my security is the Divine plan, knowing that what comes up is best for me. How can I stay connected with the Light in myself?

I walk up the hill with Susan after supper and talk with

her about *sanyas*. She says that it is what I have always wanted. I don't need to try to do it all in the next two years. Can it be a lifetime plan? This idea softens the desire but I feel sadness well up inside me. When I close my eyes I see a field of blue flowers in a sunny meadow.

For me being here is never a question or decision. Since first coming to the Ashram I have always wanted this way of life. Looking at the facts, how can I come? What do I have to do before coming? What can I bring? Why didn't the others follow through? I give up the idea of living here for now. Let it go. It clings deeply. What is surrender? The reality of this bliss path doesn't seem so subtle. It requires strength and dedication. Now the larger vision is *sanyas*, selfless service. I will listen to the guru, asking for advice. Where can I be of most help? Can I do it alone?

It keeps flashing in my mind that I've made an inner commitment to be a *sanyasi*. I need loyalty to my own commitment. My focus is offering back to Divine Mother. She gave me this life; the least I can do is give it back. Do what has to be done now. Get the divorce from Arthur, make that clear. I tell Swami Radha and the residents about my need to return to Lethbridge. It seems hard, renouncing.

Julie decides to return to Lethbridge to help establish the yoga centre. We have a beautiful talk on the beach as the sky is turning water blue and the moon is rising over the mountains. We are both excited about the future, sad about leaving. She, too, wants to be a *sanyasi* and live at the Ashram.

At the end of August the children and I make preparations and I write a note to Swami Radha, thanking her for the teachings and the opportunity to be at her Ashram. I will see what is happening in Lethbridge and keep her informed, trying to be as much help as possible.

Arriving back with the kids it's as though we're in a foreign country – the entry shock, the noise shock and the evidence that quick and immediate action is needed. The mantra and Light are here and I can feel the wave of support. I'm not disconnected but I can't overpower the sadness.

I am faced with enormous personal problems – no money, no job, big bills. I decide to surrender and see how it works. The Ashram hears about my situation and sends a donation so I can pay the gas bill. What an absolute joy for all of us – having hot water and a working stove, and that wonderful feeling of being warm again after being so chilled. Then money comes from Mom, flowers arrive from the daycare director, a Divine Mother statue from one of the swamis, goods and equipment from friends, a gift of a weekend workshop in Calgary, and a ride to the workshop from a student. The kids are being marvelous. Each night after supper they go out looking for bottles and money. They find quite a few bottles and a few pennies and dimes, and that is their allowance. They have made it into an adventure. They seem so resilient and are doing well at school. Everything we need seems to be pouring in. I have to be accepting.

Time now to apply for unemployment insurance, do a deep cleaning of the house and start my job search. But why am I here?

In the Kundalini group, I feel almost like an outsider, not wanted. It takes time before the group starts to adjust to the change of losing Susan, who is now director of Radha Centre Calgary, the first official centre of Swami Radha's work outside the Ashram. I'm happy for her opportunity but also miss her. I pick up the mood and emotional impact of change in our group. Some people are confused, some are understanding, some are angry. The electricity is intense. I feel sad and rejected. Am I so out of touch? It takes a few months to build good feeling and a spirit of togetherness. Then everyone decides I should take on the leadership.

At home I'm reading a book on divorce and encouraging Garth and Clea to talk openly about their feelings. Arthur is still living in Lethbridge and comes by to visit. They see a difference in him and appreciate that we don't fight anymore. He sometimes takes them to dinner and a movie. He seems more together, though he still has beer on his breath and is fidgety. I'm keeping my focus from the YDC by completing the thirty book reports – reading, reflecting, seeing how the texts are relevant in my life right now.

Money pours out, unemployment insurance trickles in. I'm working on dreams, talking with friends, going to groups. Julie and I are washing walls, windows, curtains, learning to unplug sinks and fix broken taps, painting. I am making the house beautiful and my own, and preparing for Swami Radha's workshop here in November. I'm excited that she will be staying with us. The house is refreshed inside and out.

The week before she arrives the school board calls me about a job. I feel clear, straight and confident in the interview and soon receive the news that I have been hired for a part-time teaching position, starting in January. Everything seems to be falling into place...

Waiting for Mataji to arrive and then seeing her I feel stunned by her beauty and her love. She and her assistant drive up just as the rice is cooked for dinner. I help her settle into her room. At dinner she talks freely about everyone at the Ashram and what is happening there. And she tells me, "Selfless service means doing something you like or don't like. It is only the ego that judges. The offering is what changes it. Make everything you do worship."

The next day the workshop starts. It's exciting. The whole group helps with the set-up, and the arrangements flow smoothly. I don't have to do everything. In the workshop I listen and concentrate. What are people really saying? I watch how Mataji gets to the underlying issues – how she is gentle with some, and cuts through and is very direct with others. At the end of the day we walk together outside, me holding her arm to support her. "Chant mantras in this house," she says.

It's comfortable having her here. She enjoys making her own breakfast and we have quiet time as we eat together. She is very open with sharing her dreams, helping us interpret our dreams, expressing interest in the children and our life here, being direct about money. And she is a constant source of stories and inspiration.

The second day of class and I observe that I'm letting my imagination run away with me, not holding to the instructions. Do I get stuck in making up pretty pictures and always wanting an experience? Take it easy, do not force. How do I surrender? I admit how my mind has wandered off…

By watching her teach I learn how she comes from a place of such care and concern, never dogmatism. I see a part of me that feeds on images, lives on practices and reflects where I am in symbolic terms. The eyes of the Buddha, which I visualize in the workshop, are like the eyes of Swami Radha – steady, consistent, full of ready helpfulness. They tell me that there is always another level to contact. How to reach it?

I can receive vivid impressions and images in my mind that no one else needs to be aware of. I can imagine Light, which is not obvious to others, but has an effect. Then the Buddha is present in my actions. This is what I admire in Swami Radha – how her actions emerge from that higher intelligence. I want to develop that same ability to really listen and speak from the Light.

Winter/Spring 1983

In January my teaching job starts and I find I have confidence in the methods I've developed and a feeling of openness to other teachers and the parents. Peace and goodwill develop in the classroom. At the same time I can't help comparing the rigid machinery of the school system with the fluidity of the daycare.

In May the principal informs me that the former teacher will be returning from maternity leave, and I won't be needed in the fall. So it's back to the job search for me. I hand it over to Divine Mother.

Arthur has moved from Lethbridge to Toronto. He calls to ask if the kids can join him in Nova Scotia with their grandparents for the summer and they are excited about it. Garth will be a teenager this fall. Julie is at the university, completing her BA. So we're all entering a new phase.

Summer 1983

How happy can one person be? I have been invited to the Ashram free of charge for the entire summer to oversee the Children's Program and to help in the kitchen. With my own children heading back east it means I will have time for an involved spiritual practice.

Such feelings of absolute delight – being back at the Ashram, meeting everyone! New Radha Centres are opening in Ottawa and Toronto and different swamis are being sent out to start them up. I feel the freedom and beauty, the love and dedication.

Today the kids leave for the east, and it's strange not having them to look out for. I'm living at Creek Cabin, the little log cabin I first saw in my dream before even coming here. I have it all to myself now and make a promise to do the

Divine Light mantra for two hours each morning. Will I be able to do it for forty days?

My first morning of practice and I am amazed. How did I keep the mantra going for so long? Guidance of the mala beads, one by one – big, little, round and round. Will it change the *samskaras*, the patterns of my mind?

What a marvelous evening! After satsang with Swami Radha I feel my body ignited in love, burning through whatever obstructs. She is the most creative being I have ever met, yet the most sensible. I want to reach her level of patience and love, and to surrender to the Divine as fully as I can. Accept what is, develop concentration, approach the voice of inspiration.

With gratitude I do the Divine Mother dance in the moonlight, my body and hands look finer, luminous in this light. I dance to Swami Radha, my Divine Mother, offering everything I am, everything I do. The gestures seem magically inspired by grace and love. They are delicate and full of feeling. Swaying, flowing, moving in the moonlight on the porch outside the cabin, I repeat the Divine Mother Prayer,

O Divine Mother,
May all my speech and idle talk be mantra,
All actions of my hands be mudra,
All eating and drinking be the offering of oblations unto Thee,
All lying down prostrations before Thee,
My all pleasures be as dedicating my entire self unto Thee,
May everything I do be taken as Thy worship.

I'm up easily at 5 a.m. The sun is shining and the world looks vibrant – washed clean, gleaming a blue-green. The lake is movement, like the gesture in the Siva dance of stirring things up. How does stirring get creation moving? It's almost like a cooking process – stirring, mixing and warming events. What is being cooked up for me? I want to stay close to the Ashram. The sun turns to stormy rain and a rainbow starts to form. The colours strengthen. It's a double rainbow, a promise of happiness.

As the days go by I miss the children. Maybe they ground me. My children are my gurus in many ways. They teach me how to be a mother. It is through them that I have developed a sense of responsibility for the creations I bring into existence. Through them I know the pangs of love, of wanting somehow to make a world fit for young people to grow up in. Through them I know the sense of commitment to something outside myself. I know the connections and the letting go. I think of my little family and then think of Divine Mother's family and how much She must feel for all of us. As a mother I have come to know that feeling, and I have come to appreciate the little things, the little remembrances. These I can re-give to Divine Mother, to Swami Radha who is my spiritual mother, to my own mother, to myself and to everyone I meet.

In the Sitting Forward Bend this morning, I repeat the Divine Mother prayer, "May everything I do be taken as Thy worship." I feel the wonder of her warm touch as I melt forward, opening and yearning for that connection. An enormous sob bursts from me and I want to run to Many Mansions and rest my head on Mataji's lap and stay there forever, protected by her love.

Sitting next to Swami Radha at supper she tells me to look into coming closer. A yearning wells up, this longing to stay here. The lake sparkles; it is so beautiful. I don't know how to express my gratitude for this place. Mataji talks about her Higher Self and how her guru is a vortex of energy that can still contact her and give her direction. Please help me determine the most useful place to be.

At the end of the day I sit in the woods, remembering the quiet, steady growth of the trees and wondering if I am part of this world of growth. I know I have found my place. I love this place down to its roots.

Sometimes my practice is uplifting and inspiring. Sometimes my body or mind resists and wants to fall asleep. Then I walk and say the mantra loudly. What I want from this practice is courage to be able to do what I have to do. I want to fly in everyday ways, soaring in relationships, in work, in teaching. I want to be a channel – unnoticeable but inwardly shining.

I am making the most and the best use of my time. Everything seems so strangely beautiful and perfect in little details. I feel an inexpressible joy in being here at this time of my life, even with all my doubts about having to be someone and do something. I am here and this is the greatest gift.

Today I kiss Mataji on the cheek, a lovely warm, pink cheek. I remember the words from my dream, "If you kiss me on the cheek, you must have your feet on the ground." I am building a strong foundation through practice.

After supper a few of us are sitting with her in the dappled sunlight under the big old apple tree. She leans over and asks, "What do you think your Divine Committee is up to?" Neither of us knows. We are waiting for indications. Walking back to the cabin I look at the ripples and waves on the lake and imagine a lifeboat. "If you ask for bread, you will not be given stones." Sincerity is my protection.

At satsang Mataji says to visualize, to feel deeply and to put our hearts into our practice. She says that putting the Divine first is hard for people who are older and have ideas of career and family. Even intense spiritual practice needs to be coupled with work on ourselves. "And," she says, "your faith will be tested. Reflect on why you decided to incarnate. Look at your situation with clear eyes."

The reality of being outside the Ashram and having to make a living, not being completely here, makes me sad.

It's mid-August. Garth and Clea are back, well but tired. I wake up often in the night, hearing the sounds of them turning in their sleep. I wonder if they are warm enough. I worry about getting up to do my practice. I am awake at 2 a.m., so practise until 4. A quietness comes over the cabin and they seem to move into a more silent sleep. I feel more relaxed. But I am still concerned that they are a big responsibility for me to look after alone. I remind myself, "I am protected by Divine Light."

The children and I talk in the afternoon, finding out where we are. They have changed, they say, and I am adjusting to the changes. I love them so dearly. I sometimes feel I cannot help them enough. Mataji's words come back to me – the best way to share grace is to give it back in kindness, concern, patience and understanding.

Victory! I have completed the forty days of practice. I write up my notes and give them to Mataji. At satsang she speaks about her own long mantra practice, and how the first time she did it, it was a matter of will. Mine was too.

The next day Mataji meets with me and says she has read my paper. "See if you can stay in Nelson." The idea, coming so directly, seems worth exploring but also overwhelming. Can I find a job and move us here all in the next few weeks? I send out my résumé to the school boards and daycares in Nelson, Creston and Crawford Bay. A Creston daycare centre responds and I visit for the interview, but the pay is unreasonably low. The next day Jo's Eatery is for sale in the neighbourhood – it's an exciting idea to start my own business, but impractical since the tourist season is over for the summer and I have no start-up capital. I try the employment office in Nelson but there is nothing.

We clean out the cabin and once again say our goodbyes and prepare to leave the Ashram.

Fall 1983

Arriving home there is a message about a teaching position opening here in Lethbridge. I go to the interview, but don't get the job. It is hard to put my heart into it. What do I really want to do? My job search continues. After a month it comes to a standstill. I don't want to be like Arthur, afraid to look. Will that happen to me? How many sunsets have I missed because I didn't open the door and look outside?

The facts are that I am going to interviews and experiencing rejections. There are just no openings right now. I think again about starting a business, maybe a teahouse? I make steady progress researching grants, interviewing other small business owners, making lists and creating menus. I keep busy and keep my mind open as I wait.

I write to Arthur about getting a divorce.

As the months pass I can't see the end to this chain of poverty. We are so close to the edge. What must I do? The spark gradually goes out of the teahouse idea; the doors have not opened.

Is this the test of faith Mataji talked about?

I want to be near her to continue my development. But I also want to have something useful to offer and renounce. I sit beside Tara, sipping tea as the seasons go by. Now it is barren. I look out as the winter light gradually lengthens and reflect on the growing times, the tender buds that somehow refresh and come to mind with each sip.

I am considering a Master's degree.

Following the Call

Synopsis of my life:

Position: Woman 43, separated almost divorced, with two children ages 13 and 10; has taught for more than 20 years. Would like work that is challenging and makes good money.

Purpose: To support my family and eventually move to the Ashram.

Where I am right now: Unemployed, collecting unemployment insurance that runs out this summer. I plan to spend the summer at the Ashram leading the Children's Program. I have enough money to cover expenses through September. Then I am enrolled in a Master's program at the university, funded through a student loan, a grant and paid employment as a teaching assistant.

University: This is the only graduate course at the University of Lethbridge and the first year it has been offered. I submitted my application and was chosen – one of twenty-five from sixty applicants. I am planning a full-time course load of three core education subjects plus creative writing and drawing classes. My program will include evening work, but I will be able to continue to lead the Monday night Kundalini group.

What this process will give: A Master of Education degree – a foundation to move into a different level of teaching, such as teaching other teachers, administration or consulting. The program will offer an opportunity to write and integrate my own experiences in a thesis investigating the theory of education. I will probably make contacts and meet many different people in the field, and I hope to be able to teach yoga at the university. I think this experience will be a good challenge to keep my own perspective, develop a more professional attitude and move into a different area of work, using skills I already have. I hope it results in a career that will give me the time and money to get me to the Ashram and support the work there.

I tenderly acknowledge this step as part of my Path of Light.

A day of knitting, thinking about the U of L. Can I do it? How will I manage – money, the kids? I bake bread, start sprouts, do yoga, go to satsang. I've completed my book reports, loving the process of study. We're arranging another workshop here with Swami Radha for the spring. Tonight Clea is up in the night with a toothache. I start to feel inadequate about being unemployed. How can I stay motivated?

They started cutting down the big cottonwood tree outside our house this afternoon. It's rotting and threatens not only our house but also the neighbours'. About 4 a.m., I wake up with a strange feeling, as if the tree is crying, calling out that its limbs have been hacked off. The energy force is powerful. I get up and knit until I can't anymore, and eventually drift back to sleep.

Spring 1984

Swami Radha is here again to offer a workshop. This time I feel myself so relaxed and open to learning. But why do I put myself down or make light of my insights? I have to watch when I do that. I've seen that my mind is a powerful tool and I need to honour the drop of intuitive intelligence that falls into the pool of mind. How I wish I could be with Mataji more often! She seems to speed up my evolution.

After the workshop we go out to dinner at her favourite restaurant in town – a leafy, open and bright space – and she asks me, "How would you like to be the director of the Lethbridge Radha Centre?"

"I would be delighted! It would be a real way to give back and this is what I want to do!"

We order wine and clink glasses, toasting to the new Radha Centre! *Om Namah Sivaya!* May the house be a lighthouse in this city!

The next day I write out my commitment:

Dear Mataji,

I have a strong commitment to the teachings and also to the Ashram as a centre of Light. I am willing and feel very privileged to give support as a Radha Centre. My house is your house. You are my family, and I welcome you with open arms and a loving heart. I will keep the high quality of teachings and will sustain the devotional aspects through satsang and my own practices. The teachings will be the focus through which my life revolves. My children, work and studies will benefit as they already have in the past.

I feel like a baby Radha and welcome guidance and instruction. It is through the practice of the Light specifically that I have felt an expansion that includes so many other people, and a desire to bring Light to them.

I want to offer back the acceptance that has been so generously given to me over and over at the Ashram.

Mary-Ann

Before she leaves for the Ashram Mataji advises me on how to rearrange the living room. Afterwards, my mind takes in the different feeling. There's a new focus, very clear. We took out the big old Sally Ann armchairs and brought in new, light stackable chairs and placed them around the altar. The altar itself has become the focal point and has been simplified to one image of Tara, along with the oil lamps and flowers. Even the entryway has been cleared of clutter, excess coats and boots, so it is welcoming and easy for people to enter. It all makes a difference in lifting the house to its new spiritual purpose.

Summer 1984

Being at the Ashram for the summer, I want to make every part of my work here a ritual – whether I'm cleaning, cooking or helping with the Children's Program. My time needs to be used wisely. On July 2nd, my wedding anniversary, I do a ritual for the end of my marriage, offering the benefits to my women friends and to women who are in need.

At satsang tonight Mataji talks about what it was like for her to come back from India with no money. Gurudev had asked her to live on faith so that people would know the Divine takes care of us. She found that she received what she needed. It's all very understandable to me now, from my own experience.

Sometimes in satsang Mataji has a look almost of sadness, as though she loves us so much that it hurts. How to return that love? The look in her eyes is like that of a servant who obeys the Divine master gratefully, and who can express her gratitude. After satsang I walk to the beach. It is a lovely clear evening with the lake still and silent, a fire flickering on the beach, stars bright and deep and scattered everywhere, and one star faraway but brilliant.

In the Children's Program, the kids work on their Life Seals drawings in the morning. Garth's shows the pain of separation from his dad. Clea's has a degree of sophistication and understanding of her own symbolism. The two of them help with the younger children.

I talk with Mataji about a tentative September opening date for the Radha Centre. Then I check with Susan and find out what I need, and start gathering things up. I'm reflecting on what a Radha Centre means to me. It is a place of direct contact with the Ashram, a place that will attract people to the teachings, but first and foremost, it is a place for Swami Radha. I want to create a room just for her, keeping it private and personal. I want to give back to her in as many ways as I can.

I remember after the YDC, I put everything in Divine Mother's hands. I told Her I would do whatever came up, trusting that it would be right or in some way that I would be an example or encouragement to others. This is still my strategy. I trust I am being used to the best advantage. I want to continue to develop my ideals – courage, compassion, understanding and gratitude. And I want to be a light-hearted spiritual person, not a stuffy one.

To keep my mind focused, I mentally repeat the Divine Light mantra and *Hari Om*. And whenever I speak out loud, I want my speech to be kind and honest enough that whatever I am saying could be overheard by anyone. I am giving myself time to ripen – "doing" all the while, but not overdoing. I imagine the future as positive and want to follow through on whatever commitments I make, even in small things.

I summarize my life strategy in ten points:

1   Surrender to Divine Mother
2   Be firm and determined – keep going even through all the moods
3   Do the Light and see it around me
4   Study and self-study
5   Do it now
6   Be encouraging to others and myself
7   Use my imagination positively
8   Use Light and Straight Walk thinking to see the facts
9   Enjoy life and know it is a valuable gift
10   Humbly ask for help when I need it

Mantra initiation has been on my mind. There is a letter saying that all Radha Centre directors should be initiated. On my Life Seals, I drew a picture of Swami Radha pouring water for me, which seems significant. I remember the *kamandalu*, the water vessel Swami Sivananda gave her, as an important part of her initiation story. But I've heard Swami Radha say over and over that she won't be initiating anyone else. I don't know how it could happen for me. To be initiated, I think, a person must have to be special, and I've heard Swami Radha say they must also have done seven years of selfless service, helping in the work. What will happen if I'm not initiated? Will I be a spiritual orphan? But I am already being filled and fulfilled by this relationship. Let the Divine take its course. I am just happy to offer our house for the teachings.

This summer I am deepening friendships with some of the ashram women and Radha Centre directors. We often meet for tea, goodies and discussion. My daily work with them is varied and inspiring. One day we make sixty-one jars of elderberry jam. And one memorable day in the kitchen, the bread rises in the oven and makes four loaves out of three, muffins keep on making themselves, and the pizza dough continues to expand and puff up – a meal where everything goes right. It is a great feeling, light.

At satsang Garth sits beside me on his last night before going back to Lethbridge to be on his own for a few weeks. At the end of satsang Mataji tells him she will phone his dad when she is in Toronto this fall. How pleased he is!

Julie arrives from Lethbridge and we pick gooseberries together and have a good talk. I'm glad she is here for a visit before going to grad school in Toronto. I will miss her.

Meeting with Swami Radha. She talks again about my relationship with Arthur and how I always hoped that he would change. She can understand that. Hope is a human quality. She says I am a strong woman and I can be a good role model. But if the strength becomes controlling, it can limit those around me, like my children.

On my last day at the Ashram Mataji gathers a group of us together and emphasizes that as teachers we need to go beyond our desire for acceptance or comfort. Her words penetrate. I know that being a Radha Centre director means she trusts me to be a channel for the teachings and to be mature enough to take a stand when I need to.

She gives me a beautiful Tara. I wrap her in my shawl and take her with me for the altar at the Radha Centre.

Fall 1984

It's the first year I join the kids in going back to school. Day one at the university and I get my student card, loan and locker. Poetry class is a bit difficult. I can see the teacher trying to build trust and I see my own self-judgement. I wonder if I am as silent as that other woman is constantly questioning. Will I be able to do it? Art class and the brush stroke technique – I like making big, bold shapes. I can see where control has limited my sense of spontaneity.

On September 14th many people come to our Radha Centre opening. Everyone looks radiant and the house is beautiful.

Swami Radha attends and speaks to the group. "You can all consider yourself exceptional people because you seek something more than the daily gratification of your desires. And it is wonderful to meet here in Mary-Ann a woman who is so eager to make her house a centre of Light and help other people. She feels she has gained so much from Yasodhara Ashram and what it has given that she wants to give back.

"It is not that the teachings are not available to everybody. They are. But one must want them. It is not important how often you come to the Radha Centre, but that you keep coming and that you keep inquiring: Why was I born? Why I am here? What is the purpose of my life? What should I pursue? How far should I go? And what is my place in relation to the universe? These are the questions that are important. Who are you? Seek some contact with a power greater than yourself, some greater Light than what is visible to the human eyes. Then you are indeed on the path to Self-realization."

And I follow with a few words. "I've heard you say often that it is a privilege to serve those who seek the Most High; and I feel that the people coming here tonight are acknowledging that there is a Most High. You are all most welcome!"

After they leave, I am alone again. A house full of flowers and a big responsibility. How will the house be transformed? How will it all work out with the kids? I feel blessed and know that we will be all right. "Radha" means "cosmic love," and what could be better?

I receive the final divorce papers, signed and sealed. I invite Mom to come out and we have a celebration. We go out for dinner and talk about women, marriage and children. It's a bonding of mother and daughter, which I felt for the first time when I was having babies. Now we are together in being on our own as women. She is alone and I am alone, and she offers her support.

I hand in my first assignment at the university. A release.

The university challenges me to use my mind, to do work that is clear and rings with my experience. I want to become a better writer, able to express myself smoothly, naturally. I finish my project for the effective teaching class; rush to art class; then to a seminar; later wine and cheese; read poetry, observe the stillness that comes in.

I dream that I can lift into the air and then I'm flying. I have a view of the countryside and I am able to see where I'm going.

Winter 1985

I see my pattern of thinking: "I have to do it alone. I need help. I'm lonely." I want to change it to, "I can do it alone – freedom, liberation." I know there is a purpose to this time of being on my own and integrating the two worlds of academia and yoga.

From the Kundalini work, I have a foundation of wholeness and a core of knowledge about how people learn, which I take to my studies. Each university course tells me something, but no one course covers the whole. So having this other perception from what I have learned about myself and how I've learned it gives me the ability to write from that whole place in myself. The Master's work is a confirmation that I can achieve something in this academic world. At the same time I am taking myself to a new and different place in my mind.

The other participants are amazing teachers and so interested in learning and life. It is fun to be together, almost as if we are grown-up teenagers. We go out regularly to our favourite restaurant and engage in animated, intelligent discussions that we carry right into our classrooms. The professors are just as stimulated because we are their first graduate group and they are learning with us.

I have one professor who won't accept our papers until she has questioned them, commented extensively and given them back to us for constant revision. She wants to be satisfied that they are sufficiently complete and polished. It is inspiring to have this demand for quality. I'm learning how to write and to carry an exploration to fruition. I do the work, but she asks the questions. It is very yogic and brings out my love of learning. The art and poetry courses balance the intellectual work. It is so good to encourage both parts of my brain.

Although it may not be apparent to other people, doing this kind of writing and thinking is new to me and requires courage. Sometimes the words I write seem so flimsy and don't properly represent the thoughts behind them. Can I think more deeply? Can I translate the thoughts into words?

Sometimes I am exhausted from working on papers long into the night. But I am using the challenge as a practice to change my self-concept, to develop concentration and to expand my mind. I am working to transform everything I do to become part of my life's path toward Liberation.

Spring 1985

Swami Radha stepped down from the presidency of the Ashram today and turned it over to Swami SP, her first woman disciple. There seem to be varying reactions to this change but I am supporting whomever Swami Radha chooses, and am especially happy that the power in this lineage is passed through women.

Several of the long-term residents have dropped their commitments rather dramatically and left the Ashram. One woman has been a friend, someone I was close to last summer. She visited me in Lethbridge a few times, and I had seen signs in her of negativity and selfishness, a tendency to make demands and tell stories. I could feel I had to be on guard around her and keep the Light going, relying on the inner part of myself to listen carefully. It was only by being clear in my own commitment that I could be a useful friend to her. Even if she rejected what was being given, it would be her choice and her path. She could look at it later and see if there was value in my actions or words. My idea of being a friend has changed to taking more responsibility, being truly compassionate rather than just nice.

In the yoga groups, if I see or hear things that don't seem true, I must say something. Each time it takes courage. I have to be secure enough in myself to be unattached to the other person's reaction to me. The courage comes from my own work.

Summer/Fall 1985

This is the first summer I have spent away from the Ashram for years. I sit typing at my kitchen table with the doors wide open and the sunshine pouring in. I am doing summer courses and teacher assistant work at the university while the children are off to Nova Scotia with Arthur and his family. I have the whole house to myself and I can just read, write, go to class, go to work, do my studies, tend the garden and cook for myself. It's a special time. I am surprised that I'm doing so well on my papers. I'm finding it wonderful to see how self-inquiry can be applied to the education courses.

This fall I offer a group on journal writing to anyone from our Master's program who wants to drop in. Five or six interested people gather and find it's a great way to get to know each other more deeply. I admire the openness of those who want to explore themselves. My work seems to be bringing out that sense of adventure, making connections for myself and communicating the process to others in a way they can understand.

The Ashram, Radha Centres, groups – I want this to be my life's work. How will it come about? What is professional in me? It feels as though my profession is to be in a group, to be a student and to be a teacher. What I admire in good teachers is their ability to remember what it was like at the beginning, when they are no longer beginners themselves. Have I forgotten? Become too confident?

I feel a strong desire to do a thesis rather than observe in a classroom. I want to gather facts and put them together intelligently. And I want the challenge of representing women – creating something serious, intelligent and worthwhile. In my heart it feels as though the thesis material is here in the Radha Centre – how adults learn. What are the essentials of learning in adult groups? What is the process? How do people become symbolically sophisticated? What are the adult stages of growth? I realize that I am a walking symbol of my own life. Could the thesis be about concentrated work, questing, questioning, listening, self-exploration, opening, concern, commitment to oneself, self-knowledge, culture?

In the longer term I want to work with adults, especially teaching teachers. If I imagine my perfect work situation, I see myself facilitating a group of people who are opening to the Light through reflection and action. I visualize a circle of culture with people defining themselves symbolically through clarifying discussions, freedom of ideas, an expansive structure, determining personal ideals. This is the way I want to teach.

Then there is reality. Where would I find a supervisor to oversee this direction? The University of Lethbridge does not offer an Adult Ed focus, so the mechanics get in the way of the dream. I decide to stay with a thesis on Early Childhood Education focused on play, creativity, language and the teachers' influence on play. As I work with the possibilities I get excited. I just need to narrow down the topic, sharpen the questions and come up with manageable techniques. It feels as though the thesis can be a success and will support all of the professional work I've done over the past twenty years.

But then I imagine myself writing pages and pages of a thesis. How will I be able to see through the words to the questions and to the real meaning? I am afraid of writing empty words. One of the professors helps me turn that notion around. The thinking must come first, he says, then you can translate the ideas into academic language. This helps me change my attitude. So first I want to find my process and then extend what I understand into this other language – taking that extra step. It all sounds possible.

On November 14th, Clea's twelfth birthday, my mind keeps going back to the moment of her birth. A new person! She arrived so quickly and easily and was a joy from the moment she was born. I felt like getting up and dancing with her. And now she's so independent and grown-up. She looked so pretty in her new blouse this morning. And me, twelve years later – after being immersed in mothering, children, family, women's groups – I am now immersed in mind, analysis and data. I never would have imagined it! This week has brought its own changes and challenges. Mind-born birthing – a joyful idea!

Mataji calls and says she is thinking a lot about me. I tell her that it's been a full semester with three Kundalini groups and my courses at the university. The work at the Radha Centre is offering me a richness of experience beyond compare. I see the expansion of Light reflected in others as we work together on the path. I will be starting my thesis writing in earnest in January, now that the course work is done. It is a challenge to use my mind this way and I am learning so much about different approaches to thinking. The thesis offers a way to translate my experiences and insights into form. I hope that it will also translate itself into a good job!

Tonight as I prepare for meditation it's as though the space around me transforms. The blueness of my sweater becomes blue light in the room – a blue cloak or gown. The room is like an old nunnery or monastery. There is a window where the mirror would usually be. I sit a little to the side on a high desk, writing or illustrating something – a book… a book of Christmas illuminations. There's a blue bird at the window yet there is snow outside and brightness. There is a feeling of warm support from many people moving within the building. A glow, a stillness, a sense of purpose transforms the room.

Winter 1986

Entering into the thesis proposal, a terrible aspect takes control and it's fear – fear of not being able to do it, of being criticized, of being the object of focused attention and differing opinions, of incompetence and lack of clarity. A pall comes over everything. What seemed exciting last fall now feels overwhelming, without specifics or structure. I am reacting to not knowing. I tell myself to keep a sense of balance. Build on what has already been done – find out what that is, start the research.

My thesis is on learning through play. I have to give myself that same freedom – to play, to question, to experiment, until it starts to come together. A few weeks later and the thesis takes off on its own. It's about finding the connections and elaborating from my experience.

I am preparing to lead a workshop on reflection at the Calgary Radha Centre next week. I will also be offering a series of seminars on journal writing to our Master's class. Am I ready? This is different from the drop-in group; it will be a regular course, part of our Master's curriculum, which I will be co-teaching with Michael, a professor who also takes classes at the Radha Centre and is my thesis advisor. My own reflection, sincerity and love of the guru are my protection. I visualize the workshop and seminars positively in the Light. I want to learn from both experiences.

In Calgary the workshop is launched and I feel calm. I am protected and the nervousness is gone. In its place is a welcoming, level energy. The whole day fits together effortlessly. I ask the questions: What is the purpose of your day? What choices did you make? Being able to practise at the Radha Centre among friends is a beautiful step. I am inspired by the work people do – the reflections, deep and insightful, about issues and concerns in their lives. I also have more understanding of the work Swami Radha has done for so many years, and realize how she has prepared and encouraged others. I'm looking forward to the seminar at the university.

I see the rhythms in my life – the high points of preparation, effort, feedback – and the low points of tiredness, the need to keep going, or start again. I see the places of expectation, of being on the edge and then the action of reworking, redoing, rebuilding. I experience the cycle of asking questions, not having answers, then allowing answers to appear. The mind doesn't get tired. What part of me does?

A day of letting go. After the last few months of work, my thesis proposal is finished and handed out to my committee. Now I just have to be patient and wait for feedback. I trust Divine Mother and the Light. I am doing the Light thoroughly.

As the first graduate student to do a thesis at this university, I'm entering into the unknown. It seems that no one really knows how the preliminary interview should go. I am up early and tension stops in my tongue. The interview is disjointed and doesn't last long. I give a brief intro. Michael says how valuable the process has been to open up study in this area. One member of the committee asks for more reviews; another asks about design; the third suggests a more thorough description. Now I'll make the changes and start the data collection. I'm over the first hurdle.

The journal-writing seminars start. I am prepared. I have done an extensive literature review that includes such recognized writers as Ira Progroff and Marion Woodman, as well as Swami Radha's work. The outline we've created provides a strong framework and the course unfolds so much like a Kundalini class at a Radha Centre. This work works everywhere! There are a few skeptics with a "so what?" attitude, but they don't affect me. It's dazzling to see so many of my colleagues diving into their own self-exploration on love, emotions, self-knowledge, symbolism; seeing them use their journal to watch their own development; acknowledging the power of the unconscious; and asking that underlying question, Who am I?

Michael and I will now be using the seminars as a basis for a lecture at a big curriculum conference in Winnipeg in May.

I dream that someone calls me and my name is "Mary-Ann Radha."

I love the way Mataji's picture glows and moves and changes with the day. Today she phones to say she wants to give me a car that has been donated to her. What a beautiful gift! I love her so dearly. And the practices she has shown me are deeply woven into my life.

Every morning I enter the prayer room and uncover Tara, light the candle, fill the seven small bowls with water and place them before Her, pray to Her, talk to Her, prepare my being for the day through Her presence. The space Divine Mother makes in the house offers me refuge. I can sit with Her for just a few moments and feel clear and nourished. She reminds me that She is constantly around in the day through Her delicate actions, surprise meetings and marvelous touches of beauty.

At the end of the day we spend more time together. I feel it is a special time to chant, to offer up my actions, to empty the water bowls, to say goodnight and to wrap the shawl around Her. For me it is like reaching up to the sky for direction and bringing that element into my daily life, each day preparing for when Divine Mother will really come and truly be here.

Spring 1986

I drive to Calgary and am warmly greeted by Mataji, who is visiting the centre. She seems fragile, older, thinner, more transparent. She tells me about her dream of baby Krishna coming with chocolate and putting his whole little chocolate-filled hand in her mouth. The chocolate, she says, was delicious. Krishna's chocolate relates to the many wonderful things that have happened to her since we last met. Have I had any chocolate dreams?

No, but for me blueberries are a special symbol, and I have had juicy blueberry dreams and a blue car dream – just before she gave me the gift of the car. I tell her I still don't have a job but I definitely have a vocation.

Back home I am continuing to work on my thesis, trying to make sense of the data. What is this aspect of mind that shapes the thesis in an empirical way?

Today our Master's program is notified of an opening at the Alberta Education office here in Lethbridge. The Alberta government is trying out interns in all of their offices. I apply for the position as an intern to the Early Childhood Services consultant in the southern Alberta district. The money isn't great and the internship is only for one year, but the experience could be a good way to lift me out of teaching and into consulting other teachers. The job interview is exciting – lively, involving and revealing.

A week later I am offered the job. I accept. I have a job – starting in September! I tell everyone! Evaluating teachers was the one component of our Master's program that all of us students disliked. Yet here it is – one of the main components of the job. I must have something to learn!

At the end of May I'm off to the Curriculum Conference in Winnipeg with Michael, where we are to co-present our lecture on journal writing. I hear other women clearly speaking on education and peace. It seems with women that the knowledge always starts in the heart and leaves the book. I admire those who are able to articulate the multidimensional aspects of their lives and work. Now I have no fear about presenting here, just the struggle to express. I find it challenging but rewarding to speak out.

I can see that the different aspects of my life are coming together. The conference is a victory for me in building confidence and presenting the teachings in a way acceptable to academics. I'm also inspired to know that others are doing similar work on themselves in their own way. After the conference Mom pays my way to Toronto to see Julie graduate with her Master's degree.

Uniting worlds, expanding mind.

Summer 1986

A nourishing summer at the Ashram, involved in groups and classes, many of them with Mataji. She is teaching us to focus on the symbolic aspects of the asanas, a process she calls the Hidden Language. What I have gained from my papers and from others will be very helpful to me and to the people coming to the Radha Centre. Somehow the benefits always sift down to those who need it.

While working with the Plough pose I reflect on having a job in a new field. It will be unfamiliar and with new people. It is an opportunity to allow new aspects of me to grow and old ones to be ploughed under and made useable in a new way. Last year at the university I learned how I could constructively apply criticism through critiquing articles and ideas. I expanded that idea to using criticism appropriately in my personal life. This year the job has to do with evaluation, monitoring and consultation. I plan to use the symbolism of my outer work to also look inward and evaluate my path, monitor my practice and consult with Divine Mother. Each situation is an opportunity to learn more about the field of the Divine. I am breaking new ground.

I try to do the Peacock Feather, an upside-down arm balance, for the first time. I see it needs a different strength. Coming out of the pose is different too. It feels strange, not part of the Hatha work I have done. The thing I relate it to is leaving the Ashram and going back to Lethbridge. Every time I'm here at the Ashram, something deepens. Then I step out into something new, which always feels unfamiliar and strange. How do I keep and sustain my connection to the Divine?

Today I visit the Alberta Education office. I feel I will be able to do it – log in my time, travel southern Alberta, do my practices. I will be assisting Gwen, the Early Childhood Services consultant, with her evaluations of kindergarten and primary school teachers and classrooms, as well as helping her with administrative tasks such as reports and research. It will be a good experience. Remember to keep things simple. What do I need to travel? My prayer rug, the picture of Mataji, mala, yoga clothes. I will start to apply for credit cards too.

My first day of work. Nervous but okay. How do I look? We start with morning coffee and I hear the sexist talk of the men. Gwen, who I know from my own ECS teaching, is friendly. She seems to know how to handle the scene and takes me under her wing. But she is looking tired as she banters, smokes and drinks coffee.

Staff meeting. I don't understand much but at least I can sit quieter than Cal, who looks alcoholic and jiggles all the way through. The secretary with purple eye make-up looks bored. After the staff meeting I brainstorm with Gwen about how we will work together.

These first days at the office feel strange. I come in and know nothing, not even how to use the complicated telephone system. My office is down the hallway from everyone else, so I'm isolated. I'm constantly dealing with guilt. Should I be in the office? When should I leave? I do the Light a lot. People ask where I come from and they are surprised to hear about my daycare and kindergarten teaching background. Most of them have been administrators in the school system.

What am I doing here? I can see I'm in a different category from the new men who are being groomed for positions in the hierarchy. Being the Early Childhood intern doesn't have the same status.

I go with Gwen on a whirlwind tour to many different schools, many different offices with very different atmospheres. We drive, fly, stay in hotels, meet principals, meet teachers. One meeting is all in French, which I don't understand. Back to the office and it's clear that my work right now is to prepare the evaluation results from Gwen's last tour. At least I know what I'm supposed to be doing.

I'm receiving good comments about my thesis from my committee. I must keep the Light going and work on completing it.

Today I drive Gwen to Medicine Hat. She smokes and talks and doesn't listen much. It's a good daycare centre with many ECS teachers from the surrounding areas. Because I am from the regional office they automatically think I know more than they do. It's a bit disconcerting! Gwen introduces me as her "buddy" and is supportive. I notice she is flustered afterward and I am relieved in some way that even with so much experience, there's still a human reaction.

I'm smoked out in the car as I drive with Gwen to Brooks. But I'm learning so much from her. She talks about relationships at work, shows me the ropes and tips me off on the political end of things. Gwen is my mentor. What can I offer? How can I be more there for her?

I move to a new office, a little crowded and small, but at least it is in the same area as the rest of the department. In this job I'm not going to make a lot of money, but I am going to gain confidence.

As I learn more about the office atmosphere I start to wonder.... It's a government office full of dead wood and stuffy old men. The work attracts people who like to systemize things. Their methodology seems to be based on threats and indoctrination. There is so much politics, so many big stomachs and smooth tongues. It challenges all my beliefs about how teachers should teach, how schools should be run, how governments should run things. Everyone seems to be in it for themselves. Many of the people have been here for so long that they are deeply invested in their positions, their pensions, their ways.

I practised the Mountain pose last night, just standing. In my job I am standing in a new place. I recognize a feeling of tension. I realize I can create space in my mind by visualizing Light. Standing still gives me inner strength and helps me see an old pattern and self-image that aren't useful anymore. I'm ready to move into newness and focus on straightness, clarity and awareness to detail. Today I'm off for my first solo evaluation. Somehow I have reached a transition where I feel strong enough to do it, not held back by fear but backed by experience. What will I be looking for? What do I see?

I start at sunrise and arrive at the school, which is spotless. But the kindergarten is noisy and out of control, and it's clear to me why teachers need to set objectives. This woman has no idea of what she or the children should be doing. Talking to her afterward is difficult. It's hard to be honest, but that's part of my job – to be straight and kind and to help set change in motion.

Evaluating teachers. I can tell as soon as I walk into a classroom whether or not it's working. Everything says it – from the way the room is set up to the way the teachers and children interact. Usually the teachers are nervous about being evaluated, which increases the tension. But the atmosphere comes through anyway.

Back in the office Cal comments on my singing. I am trying to keep *Hari Om* on my mind. Maybe I'm humming and chanting louder than I think?

Clea's thirteenth birthday. I will have two teenagers living at home now. Clea has decided not to have a birthday party this year. She is discontent and asks, Why does she have to live in this backward city of Lethbridge? Both she and Garth look forward to getting out of town and seeing their good friend Alicia at the Ashram at Christmas.

I'm downstairs alone when the phone rings, and I'm delighted to hear Mataji's voice. I press the receiver even closer to my ear. She asks about the kids, and whether we will be coming for Christmas, and she talks to me about what is happening at the Ashram.

Then she says, "I would like to initiate you." Suddenly there is no distance between us. Her warmth comes through, and I feel held by her. I am happy, surprised, grateful. I can feel her desire to give me this gift, which is so big – someone who I will be connected with forever, someone who will help me forever – that my gratitude feels small in comparison. I tell her I deeply want this closeness to her.

It feels as if I'm really being drawn into her work. Although I wished for it, I didn't know how or if it would happen. Her call also feels like a response to my desire, which I expressed years ago when I asked if I could call her Mataji. The question and response happen in a kind of bubble beyond time. I'm standing at an opening to something beyond an ordinary life.

She suggests February 2nd as the date. She asks me to write down any possible fears, obstacles or difficulties I may have about the initiation so they are apparent to both of us. A mantra initiation is the most important initiation, she says, like a spiritual marriage through lifetimes. You need to be clear from the beginning about what could interfere.

We say goodnight warmly, and I reflect about the possible obstacles. I consider my worst fears and also think about what I have learned from observing others who didn't follow through. I write:

Dear Mataji,

What could be potential obstacles in my initiation and relationship to you? That I wouldn't cherish every single contact with you, that I wouldn't be aware enough to know when you need help, that I would take what I have been given for granted, that I would be greedy, that I would allow a part of me that doesn't trust to take over. I pray for the grace and the knowledge to recognize what I have already received.

I feel so blessed to know you, to be in a house dedicated to the teachings. Your offer is supreme grace beyond what I could possibly know at the moment. I honour you as a great teacher and know it is my special good fortune to have a woman as a teacher.

My responsibility is to put the Divine first in my life.

Mary-Ann

Initiation

Winter 1986–87

I feel how strongly I want to be close to Mataji. I think of it in physical terms. How heartbreaking to know the sadness of separation, to know she exists but not be able to be near her always. Yet how thrilling to know that she exists!

The children and I are at the Ashram for Christmas holidays. I meet with Mataji today and tell her that because of the new job, I won't be able to drive out on February 2nd as planned. She says she will initiate me this weekend then, before I leave. I ask another swami about what will happen, and she says to keep my presence of mind and to give Swami Radha something precious. But everything precious I have came from Swami Radha! All I can offer is the jewel of my heart crystallized by good effort, inspiration, doing my best, devotion. I think of initiation in terms of a connection with Mataji, not as something so mystical.

It's January 3rd, our last day at the Ashram. Mataji asks me to drop by and says she will do the initiation tonight after satsang. "Come for supper and bring everything you need." When I tell her that I don't have anything worthy enough to give her as a special gift, she suggests chanting mantras for her and placing her in the Light.

I buy a card and quote St. Theresa, "I have nothing to offer Thee for all things are Thine." I offer a realistic number of practices, being honest about how much I can give consistently, lovingly and joyfully. Then I run to get my white sari and am back at Many Mansions for supper. I feel very excited and don't eat much. She questions and counsels me.

She asks, "Can you be obedient?"

And I respond, "I've heard you say that what makes a difference in obedience is the love and willingness. I can offer you that wholeheartedly."

"Do you have to understand everything?"

I reply, "No. Often I didn't understand what you were doing in the moment, but later I found out the value of what you proposed. I've learned to trust Divine Mother. And by letting Her lead me, I've learned so much."

She goes on to explain that in her experience, there are ten-year cycles. She advises me to watch whenever I reach that low point. "Stay with your commitment, no matter what. And continue to develop emotional independence."

After satsang several initiates set up the tiger skin in front of the altar. It's the one that Mataji received from Gurudev and seems to radiate an amazing power. She enters, bringing a little treasure box of powders, a plate of bread and oranges, a tiny bowl of almonds and a small water jug. She places the tray on a small table beside her. I sit close to her on the tiger skin, and the ceremony begins.

When it is over I feel like a little boat launched onto a huge ocean. I am so glad and relieved she is here that I place my head onto her lap like a happy child. She strokes my head and I feel my face soften. She addresses everyone. "This step is important in a way the mind can barely grasp. It's not even like having children, where they are on their own by eighteen. This is forever."

The smell and feel of Light is all around us. I still taste the food she fed me and feel the touch of the beads she touched and hear the sound of *Hari Om* in the air. The feeling is sweetness, closeness, love. When she gave me the *prasad*, she said, "I will share everything I know with you." It is a feeling so close, so precious, so comforting, so beautiful that I am overcome with gratitude.

After photographs, she opens my card and asks quietly, "What is most precious to you?"

"My children."

"Would you give me your children?"

"Garth and Clea – yes, of course. I put them in your care."

Mataji says someone should see that I get safely back to my room, and Susan walks me home. I'm floating out magically, not contained.

The kids come into my room and I tell them about the initiation and give them the bread that Mataji asked me to share with them. Garth is interested in the logistics and what it means in terms of the Ashram. Clea wants to know how I feel.

I look at my altar. Mataji's picture glows and I see marks on her forehead like the ones I have. I feel cooler and normal again, and pack up, preparing for travel tomorrow.

In the night I awaken with a dream of Gurudev Sivananda coming out of the lake at the ashram beach. I see a big sun reflecting on the water.

Driving back to Lethbridge the red dot is still on my forehead. As we stop for gas I am aware of the dot. I am in a bit of a daze.

My ideals are to accept the challenges and to take the risks, to express my willingness and heartfelt desire and passion for the Divine. As a baby initiate I am encouraged to put my commitment into action through the work at the Radha Centre. The moment at the end of the initiation took me back to the Path of Liberation workshop. I had that same feeling then of being a little boat on a big ocean in the giant waves of *Om*.

The red dot fades but something lasts. I teach classes at Radha Centre and no one seems to notice the difference in me. Can they not recognize the healing touch of a great soul or sense that a great saint has said, "I will share with you everything I know?" Is it not visible in my actions? It seems strange that it would be invisible. In Hatha my body zings with the newness of energy.

I have little time to stop and rejoice in it. I come back into the fray of work and classes and thesis writing. I am with Gwen most days in her smoke-filled car. She talks about what a terrible holiday she had with her friend, and I hear her expectations and what she had hoped to receive back. During the week I watch what expectations she places on me. I find the best way to respond is to ask, "What are the possibilities?" or "In this case, what would be the best solution?" I need to get a sense of the direction before I can help.

The mantra is winding its way into my mind so that now it is not just a practice I like to do, but one that is asking something from me. It is strange and new. I keep the mantra in my mind, singing it out, touching my mala with *Hari Om* on my lips. What actually happened? I don't seem to be radiating Light and energy in any recognizable way. Maybe it didn't take. Maybe I'm not doing enough. Could I be doing something wrong? Or is it just my expectations?

My birthday, February 4th, and it's a beautiful day with everything so full and zippy. I wear red. I meet friends for lunch. I will fulfill promises to myself – to work on one dream a week, to finish the thesis, to do the practices.

At the beginning of March Gwen tells me she plans to quit her job. I notice she has been wearing nylons with runs and seems depressed. As a student and intern I am learning to set things up and support her. I need to watch for self-importance and be vigilant in cutting it off. I'm finding the best way to learn from her is to ask questions. She seems most comfortable with that.

On the road again after a slow, painful day at a school. Why ditto sheets? Why every child doing the same thing? What kind of unimaginative teaching is this? Gwen says I should apply for her job. I feel unworthy and definitely not ready but I am thinking about it. I've only been on the internship for seven months. What do I really know?

Spring 1987

I have pulled the thesis together and I am ready for my final oral examination at the university. I enter the small room and meet the chairperson from the scholarly work evaluation committee and greet my advisor, as well as the coordinator of the graduate studies program. I feel confident about what I have learned. It is soon over and the thesis is approved.

The dean of the faculty writes me a letter of congratulations, saying that I have set an excellent standard for future graduate students and that he has come to respect my work as a scholar and as a teacher. Strange to think of myself as a scholar! But I have completed something that I started out to do. I have gathered research, notes, observations, and I know from my own experience what worked. I am officially a "Master Teacher." I feel good about it. But in some ways it is like walking through a paper wall and now I'm on the other side. I only wish that it would result in more innovative programming in the schools. It is so rare to see teachers using learning centres or helping children contact their own creative processes. I will do all I can to bring about changes.

Today I feel on top of the world. Gwen is supporting me all the way in my application for her position. She has announced her retirement and is recommending me as someone she has already trained for the job.

What did I learn from the internship? To work cooperatively, especially on the hidden jobs behind the scenes; that education is a business, concerned with money and is very political; that consulting requires concise interpretations and clarity. From Gwen I learned to be forthright, approach with understanding, see each teacher as a person, say what needs to be said as clearly as possible, have evidence to back up my words, develop trust based on the welfare of the children and their needs, which must always come first, treat the children as if they were my own, be proactive, aware of decisions and process and how they affect many areas. From the ongoing thesis work I learned to write, to trust the process, to relate learning to my own life, to encourage ECS teachers to reflect on their teaching situations because what happens with children at this level affects what will happen in later grades.

Today I am told that I have been hired for Gwen's position, starting in the fall. It seems like one of those miracles again! Soon I will be a full-time consultant for Alberta Ed, making a decent salary! I haven't been here that long. There are other women in ECS who are more political than I am, more ambitious and probably more knowledgeable. But I do have Gwen's support, the team here knows me, and I know the routines.

I am amazed to be moving toward my ideal of teaching

teachers. But it is challenging to take over this job from Gwen because she is the best. People love her. I had seven months with her, though, and she is generously offering to be available for advice and to leave all her files, which are in good shape, as a resource. I will miss her. She knows so much and has taught me so much.

Tonight I reach a beautiful place in my chanting, through breath and sound, an inner vastness.

Ashram, Summer 1987

Whenever I can get away for a weekend I'm at the Ashram. On this trip T., one of the ashram residents, a man I have known for many years, is apologizing for his errant behaviour. It's a tense meeting. Mataji asks him to read his paper out to the group of residents. He seems offended, as if it were a private matter, but reluctantly reads about how he has abused his management position to strike up sexual relationships with a variety of women – from students to visiting teachers. I'm shocked! It jars my idea of what spiritual life is and shows me how difficult it is for people to live their ideals. I'm also shocked at the liberties men take with women. It's a reality check for me.

I don't think he can justify his behaviour, which he is trying to do. The question for me is, Does he want to maintain his connection to the Divine and his commitment to Mataji? What is he willing to do? I'm seeing how people can be dragged away from their commitment even by their own human nature, and how that creates pain not only for the individual involved but also for the people around them who had faith in them. And it especially hurts Mataji, who has worked so hard to make the Ashram a safe place for women. Using his position of power to charm women into sex is against everything she created. She is taking a firm stand.

Mataji says there will be new rules put in place at the Ashram, starting now – no hugs, no walks with men and women together. Afterward there are reactions to the changes. Are the rules for everyone? Some people continue to support T. and he continues to be resistant. Mataji requests that we keep her in the Light. She has asked him to go on retreat, to reflect and make a decision. He could come back stronger and clearer. It's up to him. One thing I see is the fairness of Mataji's counsel.

I am feeling sad at not being closer to her. I go over to Many Mansions to help clean up but I don't see her.

This evening I'm reading a booklet Mataji has put together as her offering to Gurudev's centenary celebration in India. The stories are of her guru and how he taught her, how she listened and lived the lessons. I always remember the first time I heard her stories. It seemed so precious to be part of the listening group. As I hear the stories now, can I learn the lesson too? If I can hear it, can I live it? The stories are about telling the truth, having faith and trust in the Divine, and losing the ego to gain bliss. Can I hear it? Can I live it?

I have breakfast with Mataji. She says my time will be coming soon. And she gives me a kiss, as if to seal the promise. She tells me that Julie is making great strides in her development. She has been working this past year in California, and Mataji spent several months there in the spring. She asks me again about my marriage. Why did I marry? Would I do it again? I am not as naive now as I was then. I am still naive in some ways but not in the same way. I remember the closeness in the initiation, my head resting on her lap, wanting to merge with the Light. The touch of her was not human. It was like the visualization of Tara, where

She held me and I do not have to hold anything. I want a spiritual relationship, a relationship with the Divine, not a person.

Radha creates the fabric, weaves the events, cuts and sews the pattern, fits and adjusts it for each. Without her work I would not exist in this form. I can't stay, but I am close by her side. My heart is full of gratitude.

T. is on retreat, and Mataji is training a group of women to manage the Ashram. How difficult good management is! The women seem stressed, emotional and uncertain in their new positions. Today I disappoint them. All I do is ask a question about picking things up from town. One of them becomes very firm and says she wishes I could decide for myself because it is such a small matter and they have more important things to do. Another backs her up. I leave and go to my room. I was actually trying to help. I just wanted the question answered. I did not want a power struggle.

The incident stays in my mind. I, too, am moving into a new position of management and power. I realize that when people are stressed they create an atmosphere that is hard to enter. I see how children must feel when they get this kind of reaction from parents or teachers.

Lethbridge, Fall 1987

The first day in my new position at Alberta Ed includes a meeting out of town. I feel anxiety, then resolve. I won't take anything personally. I speak up and speak clearly. I'm wearing clothes that I feel good about and I chanted *Hari Om* for most of the drive. All I can do is my best. I know I will make mistakes and I will learn.

A week later at the staff meeting I begin to feel as though I don't really know when to speak up. I want to be clear when I do speak, and if I don't know something I want to find out and follow through. Teachers, superintendents, principals and other consultants phone me. They ask questions and expect me to know the answers. Often I listen and can give a reasonable solution. More often it is, "I'll get back to you," then I start to find out about that aspect of the job.

What am I learning? To take criticism, to be concerned about people, to be organized, to be straightforward, to use my time wisely, to accept that I don't know everything but can learn. I am evaluating classrooms, completing and checking school forms, traveling to schools to speak to parents and teachers, writing proposals for projects.

At home the kids are doing well in their schoolwork and have taken on added responsibility since I am away so much. They are becoming independent and doing more of their own cooking and cleaning, setting their own schedules. It seems as if my real work is to keep connected to the Light.

I feel as though the new job defines me and makes me into a new shape. The work demands that I keep walking through my fears.

The Lethbridge Radha Centre is three years old today. Mataji calls to wish us well on our celebrations. She is confident in our work at the centre and says we can walk alone. I love her so deeply. The group effort is lovely, and the blessings of her work shine through in the quality we put in.

I'm thinking about T. He will have left the Ashram by now. How would I feel if I had to go? What would make that happen? Not doing work on myself. But I have to admit I'm not in that position. I am honest, I am sincere and I support the Ashram.

Swami Radha has put another *tapas,* a discipline, into place at the Ashram. Men and women will not talk with each other at all, except on work-related issues, and all meals will be taken in silence. What does the *tapas* mean in terms of my relationship with the ashram residents? Will the relationships change? Will we grow into a more spiritual connection? Again people are reacting and wondering if Swami Radha's response is too strict. My way of thinking is that implementing change is an experiment and a challenge that we can all learn from.

How did this situation come about? What is my part in the process? I think back to our women's gatherings last summer. Have I been part of the problem, encouraging others to become overly social? Was it irresponsible? Is this *tapas* a punishment or a gift? I only know that whatever Mataji has done in the past has been right, and that this step must be right in some way too.

I used to envy the residents their security and placid existence. I've often wondered whether they would be able to survive in the world because they seem so coddled. I respect what I have been able to do. Now I must use what I have been given and honour it by incorporating my practices into my work even more.

I call and talk with Susan about the changes at the Ashram. We always looked up to the ashram residents and thought they would be committed to the teachings forever. Now so many of them have left. Susan says, "Maybe we are 'it'." I've never thought about my position like that before. Could we be the ones left to carry on her work? I know I can't stay where I am and I am always preparing for something more. I can't forget my head on her lap like a promise to use my mind in another way, to surrender to Divine will, to the teachings and the Light.

Right now I am bridging two worlds – my work in the world and the work of the Divine. I try to combine them and sometimes it is confusing. I am becoming more aware of working creatively and with purpose in each situation. I am providing for my children and giving as much attention as I can to the Radha Centre.

Tonight as I do the Little Bridge pose I ask, What is bridging my life? The response instantly resonates, "It is the mantra." And I am grateful for this forever connection.

Carried by a Promise

Part of my job is to go into schools, evaluate programs and recommend actions that will benefit teachers, students and learning. It is tough. Not many people want to have someone walk into their space to recommend a different approach, make a suggestion or even a comment.

I have greater appreciation for the guru who does this on a personal level and has the ability to see what others can't see because they are so close to the situation. Strength, clarity, detachment and compassion are needed to be able to say to someone there is another way. It requires great courage and dedication.

In my job it is very important to enter with the Light, to allow the space and distance, which gives me the assurance that I have done what I could. I have also been a teacher and understand that being evaluated can be unnerving, so I keep the Light going and communicate as much respect and understanding as I can.

Sometimes a group of us, who are really professional observers, spend a week together in a school. During the week we have a perception check where everyone states what they have seen according to certain headings. It is always amazing to me that each of these different people has seen very similar trends. At the end of the week we make a brief report to the staff with commendations and recommendations. There must always be more positive comments than suggestions. I can do the same things with my personality aspects – look them over from many points of view, get a rounded picture, then make recommendations.

When I'm alone on the road driving to the schools I listen to Mataji's tapes on spiritual practice and living the ideals of yoga. I find her words encouraging and attuning, a way to stay in touch and keep learning. Sometimes I wonder why I keep choosing the world instead of the deep soft mystical stillness I feel from my mantra practice. Part of me is drawn into the fabric of life like a piece of thread attached to a needle, drawn through, over and around, up and down, making the patterns of my life. The world is a practice place. It's hard to lift out of the material. My skin is losing its tone. My eyes are beginning to fail me. Time can't be wasted.

My work feels right for now – for maybe five years? Ten years? My closet seems like a metaphor for my mind. It used to be stuffed with old clothes that "maybe I would wear someday." Now it is sorted into items of functional elegance and beauty. I'm updating my self-image and gaining the confidence to act out the professional part required of me.

Spring 1988

The kids and I visit Julie in Los Angeles and have fun with her – walking the big white beaches, going out for lunches, enjoying the flowers, fruit and weather. Julie plans to move to the Ashram this summer, having earned enough money to pay off her student loans and make her commitment.

Giving the Light and letting go – that is the way for me right now. Letting go of the work and the groups and the children. Letting go of my image so I keep evolving. Garth graduates from high school in June and plans to move to Toronto to reconnect with his dad. Clea will be going into grade ten next year. I see commitment as the internal part of my path, tapping into the potential that Mataji has shown me.

Recently a swami left the Ashram, a woman who seemed so passionate about her calling and so dedicated. No one is exempt. The lesson is commitment – the commitment to stay with the teachings, the teacher and the tools. They demand a response and a responsibility. I see the challenge that is presented to me. What I never fully see at any given point is the help I have already been given and that is always available. I keep looking for daily miracles and am grateful.

Fall 1988

What have I learned in my first year at work? From my experience of speaking to groups, I've found it is better to facilitate rather than lecture, to allow dialogue among the group rather than creating a speaker and audience situation. I'm learning how to act with integrity in political situations, knowing where I stand and asking what is right thinking based on research and knowledge. Because I have some power I can advocate for people who are not yet into their true power – giving a helping hand. Just recently I recommended government grants for a child with physical challenges who so obviously deserved help to create an environment more conducive to learning.

I am discovering how difficult it is for people to change. I see this in teachers who have developed a rigid style of teaching but who are convinced that it is working. How to get them to loosen up, to understand and listen to the children's needs? Empowerment is needed, so I am encouraging the teachers' participation, ownership and involvement in the process. I stay involved too, until the doors open. I've seen for myself that an old self-image is the barrier to change, so I try to create a safe environment through visualizing the Light, listening, and at the same time being direct in encouraging change.

Spring 1989

As the seasons pass, I find my job is becoming boring, grey, lacking spark – the big bureaucracy of it all, the dullness of it, going on and on. How long everything takes! Even though I'm making what for me is good money, it takes so long to gather what I need to support the children and myself for the years ahead. It takes so long to move to where I long to go.

I have a dream that I see Mataji at satsang. I bow down to her and present her with a brilliant white rose that grows and grows and expands and expands. She touches my head.

Summer 1989

I spend what would have been my twenty-fifth wedding anniversary, July 2nd, at the Ashram with Mataji, warmed by her presence. I see her surrounded in Light, speaking from the Light, offering practical wisdom. How to be receptive like Krishna's flute and at the same time think things through?

Mataji speaks to me about the Ashram and the opportunities people are given. "The Ashram is a training ground for teachers," she says. "You have to maintain the purity of the teachings without self-expression. There is more than enough to teach from what has been given."

Mataji says that Julie is a woman whose ego took a beating from her, and who grew and blossomed from it. Mataji has invited Julie to be her editor and personal assistant at Radha Centre Victoria, where she is now living. Julie is thrilled with the opportunity.

Mataji recognizes the limitations of people who arrive at the Ashram without experience, and she works with what she is given. "But," she says, "when you come to the Ashram, your life experience will be valuable to me."

She tells me how lonely it is at the top of the mountain, the same words I heard her say so many years ago at the Women and Spiritual Life conference. Her loneliness pulls at my heart now, as it did then. What can I do to help? How can I support her?

"Call on the Radha aspect in yourself," she says. "Let your focus be on the Divine and let the Divine flow through you. Worshipping Radha means accepting all of life." For her there is no choice about whose karma she takes on because, she says, her focus is to surrender to the Divine will. She does what is asked. In this she is such an outstanding example. I, too, must do as I am asked.

It feels as though something strong is happening at the Ashram this summer. The work on the Temple of Light, which recently started, is now progressing full force. Two walls go up today. It's amazing to watch Swami Radha's vision manifest after so many years. It teaches me about patience. Ever since she was a teenager, she had recurring dreams and visions about this Temple. When she established the Ashram she found the exact location overlooking the lake, and the foundation was built in 1965. She has waited all this time – decades – without losing sight of her vision. And now, at last, it is happening.

We have our first meeting of the Friends of Radha Foundation, an organization she has set up to look after the centres outside the Ashram. She says it is our job to maintain the teachings, to protect them, to value them and to provide ethical guidelines. In the meeting Swami Radha asks, "Where have all the Radhas gone?" Her hope is that ten years from now each of the Radha Centres will inspire ten people to intensely practise the Divine Light Invocation. From there it is up to the Divine.

"Don't worry about numbers at the Radha Centres," she says. "Focus on quality." Mataji says there were six people in a hall where she once spoke but it was full of invisible presence. "Wait with faith and confidence in the Divine for what opens up. Ask that the doors be closed if they shouldn't be opened. If lots of work is done and there is no advancement, let it drop; it is a message that protects us from ambitious personality aspects."

Fall 1989

Back at work I keep thinking of the Ashram and Mataji and what I should be doing. Why am I still at this job? Be patient. I don't have to push anything away. Function from my centre. I'm maintaining my own space at work, not being drawn into any negativity. What is my aim? To feel in a centred place even when things seem unstable. To concentrate on what I know in each situation.

I'm trying to balance everything – work, house, kids, Radha Centre, myself. Feeing lonely, tired and unhappy. I know what happiness looks like in someone else, but in myself it is hard to find. When my life feels shallow, does it mean I'm not cooperating? What is happening underneath? Yet I feel very close to something – as if a veil is about to be lifted.

Winter 1989–90

At Christmas I arrive at the Ashram feeling cramped physically and mentally, and I enter the softness and beauty of Swami Radha's field of great consciousness. What a gift! Every cell in my body becomes alive and tingles. Sometimes when I'm sitting beside her something within me remembers and puts her in the Light spontaneously. Everything else is still going on but the Light is there.

Julie looks so solid helping Mataji. She has become her main assistant, which requires an attitude that she has lovingly achieved.

Mataji invites me to become part of the Ashram's board of directors. It's the first time a Radha Centre director has been asked to sit on this board. We meet and I do not feel nervous. I give ideas and also let them go. Later I help in the office, a whirlwind of activity.

On New Year's day Mataji talks to me about becoming a manager at the Ashram. She goes into details. Make sure people don't use plastic wrap in the kitchen (it is unnecessary, wasteful, expensive and harmful to our health); limit the number of trips to town (they should be coordinated to reduce gas and to work together as a community); serve up dinners (to be sure there is enough for everyone and greed is curtailed).

Why is she talking to me about these things? I'm fully employed without enough money to move to the Ashram. And even when I do get here, there's already a whole group of managers in place. How would I fit in?

Back at Alberta Ed I realize my job is to make kids happy and they're happy when they can learn in a way that is natural to them. It changes the face of my work. Could it be that the larger the vision of my work, the more my mind expands? What can I do to change this system? I begin speaking out more, and the superintendents seem to start hearing me and are interested in my ideas. They ask questions and begin to understand what the ECS program means to the schools and how what is established in children's early years plays out later.

The men at work were talking about their childhoods. Mine is so different. I remember sawdust bins, pablum on the high shelf, Mom's wringer washing machine, tubs of laundry in the kitchen, the backyard of dirt and weeds, play-teaching in the shed, sitting on the old wooden back porch. Being the oldest of eight children, I remember lots of babies...

This job has helped me change my self-image and keeps moving me along. At the opening of a new school I spoke to a crowd of 200 people – an audience of parents, teachers and administrators. I took the time to prepare and I put the talk into the Light many times. It seems important to be able to communicate ideas to large groups. The talk was not perfect but it was based on my actual experience. I was so focused that my ears became hot and I could feel my earrings burn.

Today I have an evaluation several hours away. It's an organized classroom with a teacher willing to admit her weaknesses. I listen to her concerns and we have a good exchange of ideas. It's refreshing to find this kind of receptivity, but I'm home tired after a long drive on the dark, icy winter roads.

Garth is visiting for a few days. He's studying archeology this winter at the University of Calgary. He spent last fall in Toronto but was unable to connect with his dad as he had hoped. He is a cautious young man, smart and determined, wanting to find his way. Clea is still living at home, in grade eleven, beautiful, smart, wanting to get out of Lethbridge as soon as she can. She feels stifled here.

Spring 1990

One of the benefits of my job is that when I travel to Calgary
for meetings I can stay at the Radha Centre and visit with
Susan. Sometimes Swami Radha is there too, for short or
extended stays.

Today I arrive feeling sick. Mataji is here, but should
I meet with her or not? I feel alien – this government
consultant, stressed and ill, endlessly traveling. Am I even
spiritual? But when I enter, Mataji accepts me as I am. I feel
very tired and very warm, and there is not a lot of space. But
to have this closeness to her, to see her and to hear her words,
is such an inspiration. It feels as though she emanates cool,
soothing waves.

She talks about spiritual practice – using the mind to
concentrate on the name, imagining a form so the mind
becomes familiar with the Divine, using emotions to go to
the Divine. She speaks of gurus and the people around them
and how they reflect the guru's teachings. She tells me to
study texts and to think intuitively. "Translate the words into
Light, use the Light, wrap yourself in Light, tell the body it
is protected and it is safe to go to the source of Light." She
says she does not get tired when she is talking about spiritual
things, only when people hold resentments. And she lets me
read the *Light and Vibration*[1] manuscript she is working on. It
is so inspiring!

I see her as Radha – deep, loving, compassionate. I know
she is Radha by the way she blends the teachings into living. I
see her intent and how she does everything with a purpose. I
sit listening, feeling entirely healed, as she gives generously.

Her words glide into the space between us and I am

---

1   Swami Sivananda Radha, *Light and Vibration* (Kootenay Bay, BC:
     Timeless Books, 2007).

looking into infinite blueness, carried by a promise. As the instant passes, a fragrance remains. She promises that the moment will last, and my heart skips and opens to the promise.

Summer 1990

Can I believe what is happening? So much! Jayne, who runs the Radha Centre in Canterbury, England, has invited Clea to live with her to finish her last year of high school. Clea is so excited about studying abroad. Jayne says she can offer her a room at the Radha Centre at a reduced cost in exchange for her help with the publishing work there.

I phone Mataji to tell her about the offer. She asks, "And what is your plan?" She says it would make her happy if I was at the Ashram. I begin to think one more year of work, to cover everything. Mataji asks me to visit her at the Radha Centre in Victoria. She wants to discuss my future.

I remember during the Yoga Development Course how powerfully I wanted to go to the Ashram. The group discouraged it because of the kids and because I had not thought enough ahead. Now I feel I have purposefully gone out and finalized my divorce, raised the family, completed a Master's degree, worked a demanding job, directed a Radha Centre and brought Light into all I did. Now I have something to offer. And yet it feels that Swami Radha was the source and the inspiration for everything.

When I arrive in Victoria, Swami Radha sits me down for a serious conversation. "How much money do you have now?" she asks. "Write down what your needs are and what you've saved, and what your income will be over the next while. What would you expect from the sale of your house?

Then we will look it over together."

I note money currently available, future incomes from income tax return, GICs and pensions, money available if the house is sold. Then I list expenses – Clea's plane ticket, room and board and personal expense money, Garth's university and book fees, my ashram residency fees and living expenses, plus something to set aside for the future.

When we look at it together, she says, "This is fine – you have enough here. Can you move to the Ashram by Christmas?"

"Yes!" I'm so happy!

"Your strength was always clear to me," she says, "so I didn't feel I had to spend that much time with you. I didn't need to pamper you. You do have to work on understanding financial matters, though, because I expect a lot of you."

Today Mataji helps me plan my approach. She invites L., who is in Victoria visiting her from the Ashram, to join us so she also has a clear idea of what will be expected of me when I arrive next Christmas. L. is on the board and oversees the office.

Mataji says that when I move to the Ashram I should plan to meet weekly with Swami SP, the ashram's president, to get an overview of what is happening and to be helpful in whatever way I can – sitting in on courses, being part of meetings and decisions. She says I will be Swami SP's right-hand assistant. I should look at her as my *sadhana*, a way to practise surrender to the Divine. Pray for her and pray to the Divine, Thy Will be done. "Put her in the Light, and as a practice, do whatever she asks as long as it doesn't go against your conscience. Work to create harmony."

Once I am at the Ashram I should phone Mataji regularly in Victoria and keep track of whatever Swami SP and I discuss. She will offer any suggestions from her experience. She tells me to be friends with everyone at the Ashram and to check all areas of work so that I can step into their shoes. Find out what the job description is for every person, and see if they are doing their job.

Swami SP will be giving a one-week workshop for the residents in November, and Mataji suggests I attend. It will give me time to reflect, clarify and integrate with the people there before the move.

I thank Mataji for all her suggestions and express my one concern. I wonder if she should discuss my future role at the Ashram directly with Swami SP. I am afraid I will be judged as ambitious if I come right in to help with management. My understanding of the ashram structure is that new residents go through a two-year commitment period, where they settle and take time to adjust before taking on responsibilities.

"No," she says, "you are mistaken. This is not the case for you because you have been coming to the Ashram for more than ten years. I know your dedication. It is mantra and surrender that lead to the Divine."

After my visit with Mataji, I go to the Ashram and participate in a Hidden Language course for teacher training. My reflections show me the new perspective of where I am. In the Eagle pose, I focus on clear sight and see my trap of wanting to remain invisible and unknown. But the consulting job has exposed me, made me stand up in front of others and be the innovative leader, expressing my ideas and seeing them through to completion. Many people know me now as a symbol of Alberta Ed or of the Radha Centre. The trick at work, as it will be at the Ashram, is to accept the duties and responsibilities but give the acknowledgement to the Divine.

The Corpse pose shows me that I am preparing the funeral for my life in the work world. My job has served me well, giving me an overview of education and teaching me about management, hierarchy, control, politics, decision-making, meetings and evaluation.

I see that there is a power directing my path so precisely, taking into account each detail and keeping the main purpose in mind. As I come to recognize its soft weavings into my life, my faith grows that the plan is in motion and is perfect.

I meet with Swami SP to tell her about my intention to move to the Ashram by Christmas and how I have been asked to become her assistant. I run into a fierce underlying resistance. "If people come to the Ashram because of Swami Radha," Swami SP says, "they won't stay. They have to come for the Ashram and for their own path." But this is my path! What does she mean? What is the difference between Swami Radha and her Ashram? How can I become Swami SP's assistant if she doesn't accept me in that role? Is opposition, too, part of the plan?

Fall 1990

I return to Lethbridge and help Clea prepare for her trip to England. I feel apprehensive. She's just sixteen, we have a close relationship, and we haven't been apart in this way before. Will it all work out? I drive her to the airport. A quick hug, a few tears, a few whispers and she's gone.

At work my mind is dragging with the office activities. I'm finding it difficult to be here – wanting it to be over, wanting to ask my supervisor for the week off in November, wanting to be able to tell her I'm leaving. But waiting for the moment.

At the end of September Clea calls to say it's hard for her; she's stressed. Being there is not meeting her expectations and she's unhappy with her living situation. She's used to being very independent and in her new place there are so many

rules. What can I do? Her situation affects me. I feel anxious.
I start a practice of ten Lights a day and an hour of mantra.
When I am securely in the Light I feel the protection.

I'm living in a tidy, empty house. It's lonely.

Today I get the approval for my week off. A potential buyer is
coming to look at the house, so I'm home early to clean up.
How will it all happen – the house, the group, the move? I
meet with two of the students who are also trained teachers
involved in the Radha Centre. They are eager and willing to
carry on the classes here in some way, and they are developing
a good relationship with each other.

In October I start going through all my papers and
throwing things out. The past becomes present – the divorce,
the university, my poetry, the struggle for money, the job, my
process. At the group on Monday night I feel tears close to
the surface – as if everything is being abandoned. But no –
it's not everything. It's just me, leaving. The teachings will live
on here.

By the end of October I feel the time is right to tell my
supervisor my plans. Today I look for her and try to get her
attention. She starts to talk about what she is doing and there
is no obvious way in. Then she tells me her holiday plans and
asks about mine. I say, "I'm going to BC, and there are some
changes happening in my life. It seems the time has come for
me to move on. I actually want to live in BC. I will be giving
my notice." I don't say "the Ashram," yet it seems the shock of
my leaving is enough information for her.

A week passes and I feel awkward at work. No one else
seems to know. Today I drive to Vulcan with wind gusts
at 100 miles an hour. I won't miss getting up in the black
winter mornings to drive through winds and blizzards and
forty-below temperatures, heading down straight highways

to unknown schools scattered far and wide across southern Alberta.

I wonder if everything is happening as it should. The house isn't selling and I have to stay until there is a buyer. Will it all fall into place? I phone Mataji. She says they are preparing a special apartment for me at the Ashram, so bring whatever the kids need for their room. It's their home too. Mataji encourages me to keep the move happening. "If the house doesn't sell," she says, "rent it but keep on going."

My mind is settled. I talk again to my supervisor. She is supportive of my decision on a personal level but she says it's difficult for her as the director. Would I reconsider and stay until March? It's hard for me to refuse but I am longing to go. I stay firm on leaving before Christmas. At the staff meeting in the afternoon she announces my departure and it seems everyone accepts it easily. No one is upset or resentful or even interested in what I am planning to do.

When I come home from work the realtor calls to say that the house has an offer. I call Susan and Mataji to let them know. I call Clea to check in and to wish her happy birthday. I have trouble sleeping all night.

I meet the interested buyers and they like the feeling in the house. What would be in the air that they can feel? Perhaps an essence of Light and practice? I accept their offer.

It snows very hard as I'm leaving Lethbridge for the Ashram to attend the workshop. I want to hurry but I go slowly, driving through the November blizzard into the Kootenay sun. L. greets me in the office. She seems distant and reserved, even as she gives me the key to unlock all the doors of the Ashram. This is a big moment for me – I have the key!

L. shows me where my apartment will be. It's still unfinished but it is a big suite. I want to make it tasteful, minimal, reflecting the Divine. I meet the other residents at supper and then go to satsang. I wonder if the Ashram is changing. I'm missing some of my old friends here who would always be so warm and welcoming when I arrived. Now they live at other Radha Centres or they have left the work. What is Swami SP's leadership style and how will I contribute? What will it be like to live here?

I wake up to sunshine on the mountains and a sunbeam just behind the Temple, lighting it up. I have a feeling of being uplifted as I join the residents in the Kundalini workshop.

Over the week my process in the workshop is questioning, reflecting, sifting through and infusing energy into my memories and understandings. I feel as though I am completing the circle of the last eight years. It's a distillation of what I have learned. In this cycle there was a promise, a birth, work, knowledge gained, boons offered, responsibility and a Divine Source. One section of my life has come to an end and I see how everything leaves an impact, a trail, a path. I feel in awe of the process. The mind manifests a promise and my universe expands.

Whatever I am giving up feels paltry compared to what the Ashram has to offer. My heart is singing thank you to Mataji for the opportunities she has provided through her commitment to the teachings.

I dream that I am with a group of people living together. A farm of blueberries is just ready to be harvested. It's a new field.

I return to Lethbridge to finish up my work. My colleagues know I am leaving but they are focused on their own concerns. My departure will be an inconvenience, adding pressure to their work, but nothing they can't handle. I feel invisible and somewhat useless. My supervisor seems upset that I'm disrupting the flow. I notice one consultant who has been here for decades looking at me with envy, as if he is locked in and I am free. Several others are wholehearted in their happiness for me. On my last day they have a staff party and give me a small gift. I am happy to have the chance to express my gratitude for everything that I have learned in this position, and to express my appreciation for everyone who helped me. At home I finalize my packing – downsizing to just what I will need in my new apartment.

And now, at last I'm free to go!

A New Beginning

My first day of being an ashram resident – December 21st,
winter solstice, the day of shortest light. Do I have to face
the dark night of my soul before emerging into Light? For
eight years I have waited. Now the children are grown, the
money is gathered, the experiences gained. I have something
to offer and Swami Radha has asked me to come. It's time.
I am putting down a way of life, making a new beginning.
At satsang I bow before her picture on the altar. It is as if a
gentle cloak surrounds me – a mantle – and I feel a touch like
her hand on my back. A small miracle. Although she is in
Victoria, I feel she is here.

Crisp moonlit walk – moon shadows, trees swaying,
deer paths, boots crunching, snow twinkling, empty path,
devotion, being here.

In the days that follow a weariness comes over me. Years
on hold bring forward both sides of myself – tiredness, likes
and dislikes countered by deep gratitude, happiness and
willingness. Even though I've been connected to the Ashram
for years, it feels a bit like a foreign culture. I aim for clarity of

action and thought by connecting with the Light.

February 2nd, the anniversary of Swami Radha's *sanyas* day. What an evening! My heart pours itself open, remembering her. She is so much a part of my life, such a powerhouse of inspiration. It is so sweet and precious to be here at the Ashram for this celebration. The only other time was nine years ago in the Yoga Development Course when we celebrated her special day and all the birthdays with a whole table of Aquarians. She invited me to come to the table too. That was the night she gave me a photo of her embroidered Tara – the sign that I would live at the Ashram. And now, at last, I am here. What is time and space? How does the Divine work?

I'm trying to understand the *tapas* – the silence between men and women that Mataji put into place. It could be a radical means to make women come into their independence. The *tapas* could offer us a way to change our concepts, to find out how to support our own goals, and to challenge assumptions that men have to run things and women serve their needs. The practice of silence at meals could help us focus on gratitude for what we are eating, rather than on socializing.

But why is there so much noise – the unspoken chatter of gestures, eye contact, clattering plates? Now, instead of speaking, people write notes. Are they trying to get around the practice? Does it not have meaning anymore?

Speech and silence are linked. If silence doesn't cultivate speech or listening, it is not doing its job. We can have silent meals, but can we take time to listen to each other or even to eat with awareness? Silence. Everyone has their reasons for digressions. Hard-liners bring out the guilt. What is the reason, the learning, the inspiration? If I were going to talk, what would I talk about?

I keep hearing mantra. I do my practice at 5:30 each morning and it is very silent, very dark. It seems like a violent act to break the silence. What is speech? What purpose should it be used for? The breaking of silence brings a different silence within – a focus on Krishna and his flute. Other thoughts are chanted away. Clarity of mind seems to be making inroads. I'm developing a sense of well-being.

I want to stay clear and not take on negative thoughts and keep them going over and over in my head. It's not worth it. When a thought does repeat, replace it with the mantra. Like the lotus leaf with water drops, let it roll off. Keep in harmony with the rhythm of the Ashram. How best to support that rhythm and yet challenge some of the routines?

Walk tonight. Nestled in the valley space is the old moon shadow imprint in the evening sky. Everything is very, very still. Lit-up ferry sails across the lake. The stillness lies expectant. I hum the mantra and ask: Where is the stillness in me? Why do I make the sound *Hari Om*? Does the sound bless or does the sound connect with the blessedness already there? Does it need to be sound? What other vibration can happen from mind-heart?

It's wonderful to be settled into this lovely space – the room, the Ashram, this place of practice and Light. Every day I wake up feeling indescribably fortunate. But there are also lessons.

In England Clea is feeling smothered and Jayne rejected. I receive emotions via long distance from each of them. How will the situation be resolved? Clea recently moved out of the Radha Centre and now lives in a house with two other students. The school counselor is trying to help Jayne and Clea work through their problems. The fact that all this is happening 6000 miles away really gives me the sense of Divine Mother's presence. All I can do is hand it over and trust that we are learning what we need to learn.

I have been working in the office, bookstore and kitchen. L. seems upset with me in the office and I find it difficult to make contact with her. There is also little for me to do. Although she was at the meeting in July when Swami Radha asked that I be trained in everything, L. gives me jobs of cleaning, vacuuming and mail run. My newest and most challenging tasks are balancing petty cash and working out individual phone bills through an elaborate system, which I have simplified by colour-coding.

Instead of talking to me, L. leaves notes. I don't understand this way of communicating. I can see that organization is important but it's clear to me that people are far more important. Why can't we talk directly? Why notes?

My responses to her also seem narrow. We have no interactions except for her saying, "You didn't do this" or "You did this wrong," and me responding, "Because I didn't know I had to" or "I haven't been shown." I don't understand where the lines are drawn and why I am supposed to do this and not that. Maybe my focus is wrong. Am I trying too hard to find out about L. and me? What about selfless service? What does service mean to me? I will practise doing what I am asked. When I do this L. admits her emotional reactions and apologizes. We are all learning something.

I have a new project of reviewing meeting minutes to summarize policies and principles. Reading them over is like looking back over the evolution of the Ashram. I can see that Swami Radha gave lots of space to learn.

Has some rigidity developed in the Ashram? There seem to be so many rules, limited access to information, clear-cut distinctions between new and senior residents. I wonder about the use of traditional power and authority versus intelligence and intuition. For myself I'm enjoying the freedom from the pressures and busyness of my former life, but I also want to do what Swami Radha asked of me – to learn everything I can about the Ashram and to help. But Swami SP says I should come in slowly. I can only do what is possible within these limitations.

Although Mataji had told me to train with Swami SP and to become her right-hand assistant, I keep sensing her resistance. In my first meeting with her my feet are twisted around my legs. I am tense. She starts by cautioning me not to take on responsibilities too soon. She tries to think of anyone else who arrived and moved right into the office. She can't. I am unusual. It's not at a conscious level but I feel beaten and very, very sad when I leave her. My worst fear is that I would be thought of as pushy because I have not come up through the ranks.

I look for a different way to interact with her. Instead of expecting training in specific duties I put her in the Light and surrender to what she offers, as Swami Radha suggested.

Swami SP says she is surprised I like being here this much!

Spring 1991

Dear Mataji,

It is so wonderful to be here – a constant reminder of you and your dedication to the teachings. For so long I would come to the Ashram knowing I had to leave again. It's hard to believe I'm really here and here to stay. Sometimes I miss you deeply, but then I recognize your Light and gifts through the beauty of a scene or a person. People say I am in the honeymoon phase because I am constantly amazed at the beauty of the Ashram. I've never had a honeymoon, so I am enjoying it!

The Temple is lovely! I lead guests on the weekly Temple tours and stay up to date with the changes. The dome now has two layers of plaster on it. Walking by, I often see the sunlight caught in the beams at the top, as if the Temple is already attracting Light. At sunset the other night there was a rosy glow in the sky and right above the dome a tiny sliver of moon with one bright star beside it. Going to the Temple is always inspiring and calming for me.

I appreciate meeting with Swami SP each week. Although my training with her hasn't really started, she does challenge my concepts and keeps things at the Ashram perking along. She has also been helpful in sharing her experiences of letting go of her children and extracting the learning from being a parent.

Garth is here for a few weeks working on the Temple construction before returning for summer fieldwork at an archeological dig in Calgary. Clea has decided to return from England at the beginning of May. She will finish off her school year at the local school and stay at the Ashram. The head teacher from Canterbury phoned me to say he was impressed by her determination and focus through all the difficulties. She says she learned a lot about herself and other people through the experience.

Lately I have increased the scope of my work at the Ashram to include dump run and feeding the cows and chickens. In the office, registrations are coming in for the summer, and I am gradually being introduced to that aspect of the work.

Mataji, I really appreciate being here and having the opportunity to be of service for all you have given. Thank you.

Mary-Ann

Give us this day our daily bread – my daily experiences. The reality of the world is Radha – all that is seen. What is my level of seeing?

Today I have an interaction with D., a long-time resident. He walks through the small kitchen at its busiest time, when we are finishing the meal and preparing to put it out to be served. He stops and talks and takes up space. I bring my observation to our weekly resident meeting. He writes a paper in response, saying he feels he is not being respected. Should a woman be telling a man what to do? What is it women want men to do?

The question about my relationship with men is coming up in different ways. A few days ago my back went out, and because it's difficult to get to a chiropractor from here I tried a cranial-sacral treatment from a woman resident who practises the technique. As well as relaxing my back, it seems to release images locked in my body-mind. Afterward I wrote down my experience:

I see a Chinese court. Big lions guard the chair with a man sitting in it. I am looking at the scene and the word "kowtow" comes up. I try to be aware of Light. My tongue and jaw are locked open. Kowtow to my dad. His presence on a throne means he's king of our house. I feel an area of my chest behind my heart and remember telling Susan nine years ago that I wanted to take *sanyas*. "Mataji, I am coming!" Let go of responsibility. Lower region generate Light – Light and not babies. Have Light, give Light, no more babies.

We're preparing for the celebration of Swami Radha's eightieth birthday this summer. Today I have a challenging experience at dance practice. Susan and I try to lighten things up in the class by clowning a bit. But the woman leading the class goes white and shakes with anger at us for not being cooperative. I ask that we do the Light. I will always surrender to the Light, but not to anger. We walk up the hill after the practice and she calls me pushy and says I want to get my own way. She gives examples about how I question the silence and the way she teaches Hatha Yoga in the morning. I know I do question these things. I have concerns about whether the practices are still genuinely aligned with their purpose. She says other people also think I am pushy. She is pointing out how I am perceived. Am I guilty? Am I proud? How do I respond? How do I establish balance?

Insecurity, not trusting the part that forgets so easily, not trusted by others. How I react in a tense situation really shows not only what others feel about me and I about them but also shows the inner place I have come to. Can I trust myself? Can I gain enough awareness to surrender in the situation?

I have a dream that people are asking me to reveal a past mistake. Twice they ask this. The revelation is that it was not a past mistake but a future promise.

Swami Radha phones to ask how I feel inside and what I am learning. My every cell responds to her voice and I want to fly there and be near her. She says that I am a support to her because we meet in the heart, without words.

Summer 1991

Mataji arrives at the Ashram and when we meet she encourages me to accept everyone and find the Divine in them. "When expectations are gone and the facts are looked at," she says, "there is less pain." I want to learn to let go with finesse.

I ask her about her mission and whether it is essential to know one's mission. She says it is like having a good voice – you can train it, but you don't ask where it came from. It's always with you. When you have a mission you live as an example.

I have a feeling that I want to make *sanyas* a gift for all she has done and given me. My whole being is excited and I wonder how it will turn out. Mataji also talks of recognizing Clea in some way from Kashmir, and the next day gives her a small bead mala. The mala is very precious to Clea and she takes it seriously. Who is Swami Radha?

I'm outside gardening when someone finds me and says Swami Radha wants to see me. I run to Many Mansions. She asks me to join her in the studio downstairs. She is going to record her poetry.

There's a way she does things where something indescribable starts to happen. I am sitting beside her and I can feel the atmosphere changing. She starts reading her poems. She has crystallized her learning into them and she speaks with a voice that infuses them with knowledge. They're there. I'm listening. And it's like being transported into what she knows. It's as if all her spiritual experiences have been concentrated into these pointed, diamond-sparked poems, and the teachings are transmitted to me.

I don't know what to do next! Her words and the Divine focus have filled me to the brim. When I am with her I know my duty. I leave this world. I come back and eat and sit and see, but the body is operating differently. Mind is boggled by the Light, touched deeply, allowed to soar as if someone holds my hand and leads me to the rooftops of the universe of Love. Bestowing Light and grace, lifting gently, guiding.

When she sees me later Mataji says I should concentrate less on management and more on the spiritual.

It is the end of August and the last day Mataji is here. We are chanting for her in the Temple around noon, while she rests. Then I hear the ringing of a little bell coming closer and closer. She is walking over by herself…. Light floods from my heart as I hold her in a love that is enfolding, embracing.

We meet later and she tells me that she wants me to take

care of dusting the deities at Many Mansions when she leaves, and she shows me what to do. I dust each goddess with a special soft brush, and before each deity I visualize Light. The feeling in the room is incredible. I feel as though I'm lifting up and staying there, as if I can't walk on the ground. It's very light and dizzying. There is a real blast of Light when I dust near the special drawer where she keeps the books of *lakhita*, mantras in written form, that she has received as gifts from devotees.

I dance. Go for my walk. The lake changes from liquid water to liquid light, ever changing lightness of the sky. Still orange sunset clouds reflect water sky, and the moon starts to dance on the water.

Fall 1991

Garth and Clea call to check in. Garth is still settled in his routines in Calgary, his last year at university. Clea is entering the University of Victoria. She is sick and is on waiting lists for courses, but she says everything is easy compared to the challenges she experienced last year.

On September 8th we celebrate Gurudev's birthday with chanting in the Prayer Room. Mist covers the mountains and lake, making them one. At breakfast three new swamis appear, initiated by Swami SP. They look self-conscious in their orange robes and new names.

I feel confused, not sure, uneasy. These three seem so immature and emotional. What does it really mean to be a swami? Swami Radha spoke of initiation earlier this summer, asking, "Who would you initiate knowing you would have to be reborn until they reach Liberation? Who would you initiate knowing that even as you try to help people, they won't listen or even want to change?"

What I know is that all things will work out as they should. It feels too soon for me to become a swami. I need to focus on the Divine, the work, on my own practices. The rest will come. My goal is to be here with the right attitude, doing what I have to do. I focus on doing my work with care and purpose.

I'm uplifted by the beauty around me. Fall at the Ashram is glorious! The days are golden and after the busy summer, space opens up and I have more time to do my practices. I hear the mantras in the air and feel my spirit soar.

"Your awareness will spread like wildfire." I'm reflecting on these words that Swami Radha said to me this summer. What does awareness mean? Sunset seems dark tonight, and then one big cloud lights up from underneath. Awareness – something reflected upon to see the Light within. To reflect on the day, what is the focus – erupting points of emotions or points of Light? I want to be in the Light, teach with the Light, breathe with the Light, live with the Light. Can I focus on keeping stillness and Light in each situation? Relishing reflective awareness.

Dream: A way to receive the teachings – go into the forest with a blank book. I do this two times. Revelations.

The feeling in the dream is that if I am receptive and open, something will appear. It is like a message about getting in touch with the inner guru. I bring the dream to class and Swami SP's parting words are, "If you don't know what the revelations are, then what use are they?"

Her words feel sharp and dismissive in tone, and yet the dream is not dismissed. It keeps resonating. I consider what she said, though, and reflect on the practical aspects of what I'm learning. From the summer celebration I learned that if we work together with focus and harmony something beautiful can emerge. From the work bees this fall I learned that if we cooperate, without any one person trying to do more than is assigned, everything runs smoothly.

Moon is full. After class I go to the Temple – the round Temple of Light that is becoming more complete each day... from formless to form. The mountains shine, the ground twinkles with frost, the Temple glows. Inside are streaks of light. Stillness vibrates around me. I become quiet. There is no need to move. Divine Mother is here. It is the quietness that moves. Swami Radha's picture in the centre glows, her white hair a halo.

This morning I lead a Hatha class on the Mountain pose, using the Light. Stillness manifests in the room. I feel solid in myself. "Standing still, moving toward the guru." Swami Radha will be back for Christmas and New Year's gatherings. I am reading *The Triadic Heart of Siva*[1] and it makes my heart sing, intrigues my mind, makes me realize what a treasure a guru is. It has the language of the Light that Swami Radha uses.

I walk through the snow to Many Mansions to dust the deities. The little orange tree inside is blossoming by the altar. With each inhalation, the smell of orange blossoms; with each exhalation, the mantra. I connect to the ecstasy and joy in practice and realize that Mataji trusts me to do what she has asked.

My walk tonight is brisk. The sunset is short but vibrant, filling the lake. The little wavelets carry light to shore. The sun sets behind the mountains but it isn't until an hour later that the sky lights up. Change takes time.

---

1   Paul E. Muller Ortega, *The Triadic Heart of Siva: Kaula Tantracism of Abhi-navagupta in the Non-Dual Saivism of Kashmir* (New York: Suny Press, 1988).

Winter 1991

Mataji is back! I stay with her while everyone goes to satsang. "I want someone spiritual to run the Ashram," she says. She looks right into my eyes, "In a couple of years, you will be initiating people and you will need to know a few things." Then she gives me a beautiful gold pendant of Tara.

I am stunned and tell Mataji that a few nights ago I had a very sweet dream of Gurudev. In the dream Gurudev is initiating everyone. There is a large gathering. Someone is assigned to give out gold pendants with Gurudev embossed on them to show that they were initiated. I am close to him at one point and touch his sleeve and whisper in his ear, "Thank you for the teachings, and thank you for Mataji." He smiles and hugs me. His eyes are very brilliant. He radiates.

It is as if the pendant has come through the intangible dream realm from Gurudev to Mataji to me – from formless to form. It is precious beyond imagining, a confirmation.

It's December 21st – exactly one year since I arrived.

Guru Devotion

Dark stillness penetrates the living, breathing Temple. I sit
with quietness, mantra, breath. Gratitude is abundant like
space. Light waves down through my body. I am preparing.
I call to Mataji, "I am here!" The response is waves of
Light, and I focus on breathing to the same rhythm as the
Temple itself.

I ask for my ancient self to become present so I can do
what I need to do for Mataji's work. I know it will happen
when it needs to.

Hearing, in the silence, the little prayers going up.

The residents gather and reflect on the question, "What
kind of person do I want to be in 1992?" I want to be more
positive, straightforward and able to use the critical mind to
analyze events, decisions and actions. And to overcome being
critical of myself.

Reviewing my first year at the Ashram I worry that I am
not accepted or have not earned a legitimate place here. I trace

the feeling back to being the first of eight children. My parents were married in September and I was born in February so my early arrival was likely a contributing factor to their marriage. As a child was I overly responsible to compensate for being born? Arriving ahead of schedule, causing disruption, then criticizing myself and asking, Do I have the right to be here?

My practice is to substitute Light for criticism. It reminds me of dusting the deities at Many Mansions. When I bring in care and attention the underlying beauty reveals itself. When the dust is removed what is underneath shines. When I am not critical I am naturally joyful.

Resident meeting. Feeling of not belonging, of being reprimanded. "I don't know why you are thinking that way. You must be clear in your thinking and not jump all over the place. Only if two people make leaps in the same direction can something happen," Swami SP says. But I remember brainstorming in other groups and it seemed to work. Egoless – what does it mean? What are opinions? Do I have a right to mine?

I think back to teaching this morning's Hidden Language class. I have a fierce conviction that my role as a teacher is to ask the questions and allow the students to discover their insights through reflection. It's not up to me to make corrections or manipulate their bodies into the perfect pose. The impression from my colleague is that I didn't do it right. I feel as though I'm bumping up against unstated rules, a certain way of doing things that doesn't seem like Mataji's way. How can I trust the process here? Sometimes it feels linear and superficial instead of heartfelt and deep.

A call from Swami Radha. She asks about my dreams and says that dreams will tell me what I need to know in a way that I can accept.

I dream of being at an old workplace, unable to communicate.

How can I deepen my understanding and communication? Through clarity, intensity, envisioning, concentrating, experiencing, making connections, weaving ideas together, crystallizing thoughts – a diamond approach.

Alone tonight in the Temple I remember how I grow into a pose by doing it. I need to grow into my position here by doing it. The Temple is very quiet. My breath becomes even, and the Light comes and storms my mind. I see Mataji in my heart.

There has been a decision not to send a card to Mataji or celebrate her *sanyas* day with a *puja*. Instead they will send a fax. A fax? It seems silly! What is worship? There is wrong action and I know what it feels like.

Mataji phones. She invites me to come to her new house in Vancouver for a week in May as part of my training. I hold the news warmly within. If I do the Light ten times a day for 100 days, I will have 1000 Lights to support my surrender to her. Sitting in the Temple the chandelier lights reflect onto themselves in an endless progression into the night.

February 2nd, Swami Radha's initiation day. I'm up early to chant for her. Supper meeting with initiates. Sari, satsang, fax.

I re-read my papers from workshops and classes with Mataji. They are incredible – so deep and rich. It feels as though the work we are doing now is skimming the surface. Why? What is missing? I want to know. I think of my co-teacher commenting on my Hatha teaching, "Why don't you follow the book and stop bringing in your own experience?" If we don't use our intelligence and experience, how can the teachings come alive? Do we just "go by the book" and forget intuition? Doesn't that lead to institutionalized learning instead of encouraging people to find what they know through personal experience?

A few days later Mataji calls and extends my time with her to a month! She says I have common sense and can surrender to her instructions.

Tonight the Temple is absolutely quiet as I do the Light. It is as if I am grabbed by the Light and dance with it.

Vancouver, May 9 – June 3, 1992

I am thrilled to be here with Mataji and she is pleased to see me! My dream the first night is two words, "guru devotion."

The first few days I am in training for when Julie leaves for California to attend a book fair and offer workshops. I learn to help with showers, massage, cleaning, preparing meals, shopping, fixing flowers, gardening, correspondence. Mataji is constantly involved in the happenings of others – phone calls, faxes, letters, business. The days go quickly.

I feel a bit scared when I start looking after her on my own. But I know I will be fine because it was my inner calling that brought me here. It must know what to do. And she is also very clear about her needs, which helps me.

I try to keep my focus on Mataji – loving her the whole time, keeping her in the Light. She naps. She reads voraciously much of the day and is involved in the *Light and Vibration* writing project. I drive her, trying not to be too jerky. She talks about using every opportunity to teach. My other life seems to fade.

Sometimes in the day I mentally affirm, "You have access to all of my mind." I sit and hum and think of nothing in particular, and then something happens – a softness in the room, or a certain look comes over her, or ideas arise. Why did you marry? she asks again. I continue to explore my motivations.... Why did I?

We talk about the Ashram. She has a concern about the Yoga Development Course. What is the emphasis of the course? What is it that we want people to come away with? She feels that if graduates from the YDC want to teach, they need to do more than just the three-month course. The idea behind writing the book reports is not just that students read original texts on yoga, but that they apply what they've learned to their own lives. We should also be more demanding, firming up the timeline for completing the reports to one year and asking students for a clear focus on one subject. How can we assess whether we are actually training people to use their intelligence and discrimination? We don't want to encourage theoretical learning. How much do graduates from the course understand the teachings and symbolism? Can they see their own self-development? Perhaps they could be evaluated in another way, by presenting a talk on what yoga is or by writing an essay on each one of the yogas, using their own bibliography and personal experience?

At the Ashram I am an outsider to this kind of exploration and decision-making. I write down her ideas, fascinated by how she approaches from so many angles.

She advises me not to be too busy with the day-to-day work of the Ashram but also to balance it by focusing on the bigger world we live in.

Swami Radha is always up each morning completely fresh, happy, bright and eager. Today she is involved with brainstorming possibilities for this new house in Vancouver. She is still unraveling the facts. She seems excited and involved in figuring out alternatives for the house if the people who plan to move in do come – how it will be a Radha Centre as well as providing some rental income. But if they decide not to move in, how would she manage financially? What would she do with the space? She generates a list of options. I am learning from her example of keeping detached and thinking through alternatives.

I help her as she sorts out where everything should go in the house. She works, steadily focused until each area is tidy and the items are easy to find, creating space, too, for the people who may be moving in. She just keeps going. She doesn't mind putting things in one place and then rearranging them later. Each object must be in the right place for practical purposes and for esthetics. I love this day.

I will do anything for her, not always perfectly the first time. My day is 8 a.m. until 10 p.m., no break. Full moon shining in my window and I sleep right through it.

One day she barrages me with questions: Where does your process of thinking get the energy from? How much energy do you use to produce a sentence? Is the energy of your mind different from the energy of your body? What is the difference between emotions and feelings? Can you drive the intellect to a point where it won't answer anymore? Then what happens? What is the energy of the mantra? Why would it be self-generating? Generating what? Does it generate energy? Is this the same energy that is used for thinking? Would I have more if I didn't think of anything but the mantra?

I remember sitting in the Temple and how the sacredness of the space affects my mind and the silence affects my breath.

Sitting next to her – her eyes are warm, her ways of doing things straight on. I keep my own back straight so the energy will move straight up. Mataji talks of letting go of what has been placed on us and taking back what is our birthright. I've seen this happen in my own life when I accept a challenge or make a commitment.

I love her and want to be a *sanyasi*.

Another disciple arrives and his ongoing presence takes

over the space and the focus. The expectations of discussing *sanyas* have to be put away. I will wait. What is the big deal? I have come to serve, and that I will do willingly and good-heartedly. Each night Mataji comes in and says goodnight and a kind word.

I dream that Mataji appears walking up and down the stairs, showing us how agile she is. Then she walks on the road and doubles over and becomes a white triangle. Julie picks up the white triangle and puts it into water and it becomes Mataji again.

The triangle is powerful, like her essence. The dream seems to reveal how she keeps coming back for us, how we will recognize her. In the Sakta texts, the triangle represents the feminine and is symbolic for action, will and knowledge.

Sadness that my time with her is up. Sadness about not asking for *sanyas*.

Summer 1992

I return to the Ashram and send Mataji a poem about my time with her.

> *Sacred Time*
> The past and present stopped   looking into eyes
> that are not speaking of now or later or future or sometimes
> She is speaking of always
> and waiting for it to happen now
> The orchid placed away from the window
> returns to the window's light   once there
> the blossoms continue to come
> and last and last and last

I join the Temple Dedication committee and we launch into planning and preparation for the celebrations in mid-July. Who is to do what and do we have enough of everything? So many people are coming that we book extra accommodation outside the Ashram. The grounds are being spiffed up and we are learning new *bhajans*. The Temple itself is receiving its finishing touches – final coats of paint and varnish, topsoil around the building, installation of the Divine Light flame in the reflecting pool. There is an air of palpable excitement. And as always, a few problems arise.

The woman organizing dance practice says she is frustrated because she wants the outdoor dance platform carpeted. She has spent several days researching carpets and the decision needs to happen right away, she says, because the platform will be too hot for the dancers, who will be barefoot, between noon and 2 p.m. I point out that the emphasis of the celebration is on the Temple, and the work force is focused on completing it. Also the schedule is made up and we will not be outside in the sun during the hottest time of day. Another board member says that the kind of carpet she is suggesting is slippery, especially when wet. The dance organizer brushes aside all of our concerns and suggestions, saying she has already thought everything through. In the end we decide not to do it.

I remember Swami Radha putting in time and effort to think things through, but that was only part of the picture. The other part was detaching from the outcome once the research had been done. This situation gives me insight into the process of the Ashram, the committees and the responsibilities. I need to maintain an overview while working on day-to-day events. I need to be able to say no if it is for the greater good of the Ashram. Again it seems such a privilege to be here involved in this ongoing learning.

Reflecting back on my time with Mataji I realize something intangible happened there. Because I was concentrated on a variety of work my focus was not on the work itself but on the guru and wanting to serve. Although it's a subtle shift, I recognize that feeling now when it's happening.

L. returns from her travels in eastern Canada. She enters full force and I feel shaken in the wake of her negative remarks and criticism of mistakes. How can I maturely handle this difficulty in communication between us? I can't take everything personally or get caught in thinking what I think she thinks. How do I step out of that? Become aware of making a choice from my strength – not the limited child but the mature, thinking adult and seeker. My practice is to own the mistakes, not react, let the comments be, make the corrections.

I think of L.'s tendency to stick to the letter of the law and her desire to be the leader of the group, and Swami SP's desire to be the mother of the group. Where is the inspiration? How does one call on Mataji and believe she is really here? How do I? What is meditation? What is the Light? Do I really desire it?

Today we have a good meeting that includes Don G. He's a long-time disciple who lives away from the Ashram right now but often advises Mataji. I can see he isn't afraid to think and be practical and expand beyond the usual boundaries. The vision of the Ashram that we two could generate would be phenomenal! It feels as though something is just starting to come into being and define itself.

Friday – the first night of the Temple Dedication celebration. It's warm and summery and the Temple is filled with people. The inner lotus doors close and Mataji enters through one of the seven glass doors. She is wearing a most delicate white silk sari, and stops, slips off her shoes, then *namastes* with loving eyes to everyone. Sitting, she leads us in chanting *Om*, which

reverberates throughout the space. Then she speaks of the
Temple as being built in the unseen, a symbol for the Light
– the eternal part in us, the uncreated, the undying. She leads
us in seeing the Light flow into the body and settle in the
heart, so that the heart is filled with Light. "That," she says,
"is the state of perfection." We repeat the Light mantra and
chant for her. It feels as though we are inside her living vision.

Saturday – guru *puja* in the Temple, an opportunity to
prostrate before Swami Radha and offer her rose petals as a
symbol of gratitude. My heart pounds, opening to the Divine
force she keeps giving out. I can't wait. I want to jump up and
tell her how much I love her. Letting the Light flood in and
fill my heart and my being. Shaken. Shaking in the Light. As
I bow before her I clear away some rose petals and containers
so there is room for everyone. Being of service while my heart
pounds and the fragrance of roses wafts up.

How does the Light come? How does it make itself
evident? How do I receive it and share it? How do the
teachings come through? Over the three celebration days I
serve, and it is service that makes the teachings clear and real
to me. I take care of the needs of the people, organizing and
being accommodating enough to look after whatever comes
up. I need to be brave, focused and open. This is the training.

Temple, guru, rose petals, people, devotion, service – one
foot in heaven and one on earth.

Today I have to go into Nelson for day surgery at the hospital.
I am asked the routine questions as I register. "Where do
you work? What do you do? Who is your next of kin?" The
questions seem so oddly out of context, and I wonder what
my reality is now. How do I connect? After they prepare
me I'm rolled down the corridor to the operating room.
Disembodied voices. Out like a light. As I'm coming to, a

nurse asks, "What are you so worried about?" I try to say, "I have to take *sanyas*," but my mouth is very dry and the words won't come out. I am given water and a warm blanket.

Sitting with Mataji, I smell the marigolds on my hands from arranging them for the Temple. I tell her about my experience coming out of anesthesia and the words from my unconscious that I have to take *sanyas*. She says that *sanyas* is not essential for me right now. But she repeats that I will be working closely with Swami SP. "You have the vision and must compliment the narrowness." How to protect the Ashram? It is a stormy night. What is causing the storminess?

I meet with Swami SP. She spells out her strategy for training me as her backup and invites me to become part of the management group. Then she immediately calls a meeting of all of the residents to announce the changes. I'm surprised that she is being so up front about everything. Most residents are also surprised because up until now there was no indication that I was being prepared for this position. Did Swami Radha speak to Swami SP about taking quick action with my training?

So it goes – very similar circumstances to my time of transition at Alberta Education. I have similar questions to myself too. How did I arrive here? Will the others accept me in this position? It feels as though I am in a process of intensive immersion.

At the end of August, Swami Radha leaves for the Radha Centre in Spokane, where she will be staying. I have a deep sense of gratitude and am touched by her trust in me. This week I have been cleaning and straightening the Temple. It is filled with the smell of marigolds – pungent and penetrating – a smell I love. It reminds me of my first Life Seals, and the garland of marigolds that symbolized my attraction to the teachings.

When Mataji is gone I notice some reaction to the

new direction and to my training. In the management meeting Swami SP talks about people from the past who did not complete their two-year commitment but were given positions of responsibility, how they craved power and thought they were special because they were "Swami Radha's people" and above the others. It seems pointed and hard not to take personally.

I can see that Swami SP is tired after the summer, and I'm concerned that she thinks Swami Radha will be directing my work. She must see me as a threat instead of a help. I ask to speak to her and clarify that I am to be trained by her and report to her and help her in any way I can. I don't know what it will look like but I would appreciate whatever she can give. When I think more about it I suggest that I write a weekly report of what I see happening at the Ashram and include questions that come up for me, which we can then discuss. I know questions worked best when I was learning from Gwen at Alberta Ed. She agrees to this approach.

I feel hopeful that we can work together. I know from my government job that when I was hired for the consulting position without going through the usual channels it created waves. I learned a lot about hierarchy from that experience. I'm hoping it can be different here, that we can work together with willingness and cooperation. I am keeping Swami SP in the Light. I trust that this is all Divine Mother's work, and I am willing to do whatever I can.

Fall 1992

In September during the quiet period, the residents meet for a workshop. My reflections are about skipping ahead. I remember myself as the young child who skipped grade two. I get out the old photo album and find my pictures in grades one and three. I am wearing dresses that my granny made, and my hair is tightly braided. The feeling of that time was of making a leap, being out of my depth, being with big kids who knew the routines. They would sit together with their friends and I would be alone, trying to figure out what was going on in this new classroom. I remember doing so well in grade two – the feelings of accomplishment, finishing the pages, being able to read. Then halfway through – the change. How did I deal with it then? A hiding feeling – hiding the fact that I had done well and hiding the fact that I didn't know. I wanted to disappear.

It seems that the incident so long ago is part of what keeps happening at each transition – my promotion at Alberta Education, my taking on the leadership of the group in Lethbridge after the YDC, and now again skipping ahead to a position of responsibility at the Ashram. The child did not make the choice or have a part in the decision. Now I do. Surrender to the changes has a conscious element – the decision. I can see the facts clearly and do the best I can. I can learn. I can use my past experiences.

I was asked to come to the Ashram to help manage and to be Swami SP's right-hand maiden. At first it seemed a distant, eventual thing. Now it's happening – not quickly, but in bits and pieces and will continue to happen. It has to do with Swami Radha's trust in me and with my sincerity and commitment. It is awesome and scary.

I've been reading the *Radha* book[1] and finding it helpful to hear about Swami Radha's struggles and doubts and also her victories. I am trying to figure out how to be with Swami SP. Many of Mataji's experiences of learning happened when she was with Gurudev, and the actions were

---

1   Swami Sivananda Radha, *Radha: Diary of a Woman's Search* (Spokane: Timeless Books, 1981).

a basis of the teachings. Would it be helpful if Swami SP and I had some time together? I tuck the idea away, wondering if that would ever happen because it doesn't seem to be her approach. But the very next morning she asks me to come with her to Lethbridge for the opening of the new Radha Centre there.

It is wonderful for me to be back in Lethbridge to see the commitment of the group after almost two years on their own. Something precious was passed on and they have recognized it – caring for the teachings and for each other. And it is also good to be with Swami SP outside the Ashram. On our drive back she talks to me of how the powers are generated in our speech and how we have to step forward to other levels in ourselves. I appreciate this wise part of her.

A weird sadness overtakes me and I want to be near Mataji. I suppose it's the incredible lack of clarity I get caught in, like a mesh around me. The office often feels like a battlefield. The more responsibility I take on, the more aloof L. becomes. It is as if she resists letting me know what is happening. I also don't really know what she does. What is she responsible for? How can I learn from her? By following her around? But she doesn't want that. She disengages. Why? Control? How does she talk to people? What about? Where does she get her guidelines? Who does she check with?

L. and Swami SP are both sick. It seems to me that L. uses her frequent illnesses to disengage from the work and people. What is it I want to say to her? How do I want things to change? Is she afraid of me? I find she protects herself so much that it must be hard for her to develop trust in the Light. What is the compassionate thing to do? I decide to tell her the effect her sickness has on me, the office, the work and other people, then listen to what she has to say. Is there something she can learn from me also? But why would she want to?

I want to face situations straight on. What am I willing to sacrifice? "Thy Will be done." Do the Light and put it into action.

L. seems distant today, but I go through with my plan. We engage. "Are we on opposite teams?" I ask. She tells me that the office work is not challenging for her anymore. She is willing to let me do more of it so she can focus on creative projects. A year ago, she says, she would have been threatened by me but now she isn't. She wants to show me what she knows. I know I can learn from her but I definitely don't want to exercise her degree of control. She says she will write down the elements of the job.

Tonight there is a full moon over the Temple – brilliant as a pearl in the ring of mountains, glittering smoothness on the lake. I'm walking as if in a black and white film – everything is light and dark but without colour.

In November, Garth and Clea both come for a visit. Garth has just turned twenty-one and Clea will soon be eighteen. I wonder if they can truly act on their own. Did I teach them to fly? How can anyone make someone else into something? I feel it's only by example that we lead. I want my children to be able to live without the pressures of being judged right or wrong. I want their idealism to blossom. How do I accept their limitations? And how do their situations change without my interference?

Part of the duty toward my children was to raise them. Another part is to let them go. I know I have personally gone through stages too, and I have seen others go through them. I need to keep a more compassionate view of Swami SP. Is her resistance to training me just a stage? Perhaps she thinks she is too old to be president or maybe she is afraid I will take over and do too much. I just don't know. How is my training with her supposed to happen? She has talked about it and announced it, but she doesn't act on it. I also have a hard time when she speaks negatively about Mataji, as she did in the last management meeting.

Sometimes I'm frustrated. It feels as though this is a time of gathering until understanding ripens. I once heard a native elder describing consensus as an understanding of the group. No one gives up their view. We just come to a point of understanding until we agree. Can we do that? When we give up our individual duties and desires in order to serve the bigger work, there is clarity. Then others are attracted and the work spreads. It is really about renunciation.

I ask for a dream about *sanyas*.

I dream that I am going in a boat across the water. Blue blanket. Moon shining. At times the waves are high. Moon goes behind the cloud and it gets dark. We go down into a space of brilliant light and a green meadow. An elder-chief-medicine-man stands on a rock face as an Eagle with feathers and an eagle mask, saying, "Jump!" to me. I, too, am an Eagle. Consensus.

At a management meeting in December I'm told that I will become the program secretary and L. will be my backup. That's a twist! The program secretary is a full-time job of keeping track of registrations, organizing courses, working with people. I am very enthusiastic about the opportunity. Working hard and from a place of trust I do more today than I have ever done in the office before. L. is training me in setting up the Christmas and YDC programs. I am in transition and am still threading together what the job entails.

In Hatha I look at the situation through the Twist,

starting from a firm foundation, looking back to the past, then bringing what I know forward into the present. Each time I do the Twist, it is more open and I can see further behind me, seeing the circumstances that have brought me to the present moment. As I work with the pose, I stay longer and go deeper and become more open. I feel open to the work. I don't know everything but I will try my best.

How do I worship my guru? Do the work, which extends the spiritual elements into my life. Through the work I give back and then I seem to receive even more than I give, in an endless round of gratitude.

Winter 1992

December 21st, and my first two years of residency are up. Is there a decision to be made? Staying here or going back? Back to what? The choice is clear to me, and a few nights later we celebrate my residency commitment with a party. I want to read from the *Radha* book. Swami SP tries to discourage it but I am connecting with this passage.

I read from Swami Radha's time in 1955, when she was at Sivananda Ashram in India. "Here in this holy atmosphere one cannot help but remember, in one way or other, one's real Divine nature. This love I feel now is the reflection of all those who have spent their time with me, helping me. I have found myself a member of a holy family. Holy and happy. Yet they are people like any other. But what awakens this love is their own love for God, to be one with that. What makes them all so loveable is their sincere struggle, their longing for the Divine, visibly expressed in the love and devotion to the guru."[2]

---

2   Ibid., 149–50.

I comment that I, too, have had my struggles and I can see that others do too. But my experience is that the Ashram and Swami Radha's work is more precious to me than anything else in the world. I feel privileged and fortunate to be here with everyone, working on myself in this place of Light. Swami SP looks at me as if she really sees me. There is a warm feeling in the group and everyone joins in the discussion, talking about why they are here and what living at the Ashram means to them.

There is so much snow at the Ashram this year – fluffy, white and up to the handrails on the stairs. I'm out shoveling when I suddenly feel a very sharp pain in my back, a disconnection. My back is out. I go to a chiropractor in Nelson and learn that one of my lower vertebrae is fused to the sacrum. When pressure is applied the muscles tense to support and protect it. Then an adjustment has to be made.

Maybe in this new position of program secretary I think I have to do everything myself, and I am not even sure how to do it all. I've been putting myself under pressure. I took on the shoveling because other people had sore backs, and here I am! But my back is teaching me something. Instead of taking all the pressure, I can delegate.

I need to give myself time to "adjust" and make the transition. With so many people coming, the winter conditions and the scope of the work, I feel as though the fragility in my back reflects my emotional condition. But I am taking time, finding ways to adjust, to straighten out my thinking, and to make the best of the situation. I work to capacity from a standing position, then withdraw to a quiet place to lie on my back for a short time. It seems to increase the healing and reinforce a new pattern of using time wisely instead of going along with a routine.

I like moving in this new direction of coordinating and delegating rather than being overly responsible – a sense of cooperating as a team rather than being the one who does it all. It's freeing and seems right for the Ashram.

During a cranial-sacral treatment, another message arises. I see Gurudev and he says I have promised something and that is why the marriage and divorce, the ability to bring my children to the Ashram. I have promised.

And I whisper in his ear, "I will keep my promise."

The Presidency

January 3rd, my mantra initiation anniversary. During
my cranial-sacral session, I see Mataji and me in the high
mountains in a cave by a fire – warm. All of the world outside
is mountains and snow and a brilliant sky. I promise I will
remember her forever and she gives me an initiation.

How does the body release these images? Are they scenes
from the past? The images of Gurudev and Mataji give
me a different feeling of security. They seem so healing in
themselves and I often just rest my mind on them in the
quiet times.

What is reverence? Acknowledging the Light, acting on
and listening to the Light. To be reverent is to take a
stand, not letting things slip by, being brave enough to
mention concerns and bring them into the Light. I
want to respect the part of me that desires transparency
enough to take action. Explore what has taken place,
the impact, the misunderstandings, bring situations

to a clearer place so they are not left unresolved.

I need to ask for more information at the management meetings. What really are the priorities? How do things operate? What is people's work? What exactly is my job? Do some people just do what they like? Is teaching done by formula now, instead of by individual? Is there only one way to teach? What are we giving to people and what are we protecting?

We have to think things through, taking time to get perspective and clarity of purpose. If an area requires change, we can watch how people respond and give them a chance to present their ideas and express their doubts. I see that rules can't stand on their own for long. Another level of care has to come in. We need to build on our awareness, not on rules.

People here need to become more flexible too, in their work and teaching. I want to get to the core of things, as Mataji does. Keep the essence but make the leaps.

In my reflections I have been noticing two personality aspects based on what I picked up from my parents. I call them "powerful" and "pathetic." Powerful – the man, the father of the house. Everything was powerful about him. His word was the law. He ran and organized the life of the house in terms of rules and money, including how much money my mother had, what she was given and did, even how she looked. Pathetic – the situation of my mother – not able to do much, limited by the house and kids, the dependency. She describes herself as not knowing her abilities or talents; a lack of opportunity.

How do these two play themselves out in my life? Powerful says, "I have to do it, the family, the livelihood, everything depends on me. Given my responsibility this is what I must do." Pathetic says, "This is what I can't do, how would I ever do it? Why me? What is happening?"

If I look at my work situation at Alberta Education,
women who had powerful positions became the target of the
powerless women who felt unsupported or lacking. Their
excuses were put out as blame onto others. And powerful
women didn't want to assume power because it made them
responsible.

This evening Swami SP's voice rings out in a tone –
challenging but indirect. Her tone reminds me of my mother
when she would take a powerful stance by putting someone
else down. When she speaks this way about me I can see I
react by becoming the pathetic one.

I don't want to function from either extreme but from
my centre. I am observing myself and learning to name the
emotions, note what is happening, understand the point
and let it go. I don't agree with the "us" and "them" attitude
that the ashram leaders take toward the Radha Centres and
Timeless, the publishing branch. It creates an unnecessary
sense of separation. But if I identify with the Radha Centres,
then I'm emotionally hooked. It's when I become emotionally
hooked – even if it is identifying with something that I feel
is positive or good – that I seem to get caught in the pathetic
image.

To counteract the tendencies, I am practising "I am
functioning from my centre." My responsibility is to follow
through, to think for myself and to investigate what is
underlying my own tone as well as my reaction to others.
It takes courage to own my ideas and stay in touch with
my inner process instead of trying to please someone else.

In the office, I am making a list of everything I do to get a
sense of the dimensions and details of the job. My plan is to
give it to L. so she can add anything further; then we will go

over it together and come up with my job description.

I am missing Mataji's presence. I am sad because it is almost February 2nd and I haven't taken *sanyas* yet. I chant in the Temple, come to the office and the phone rings. It is Mataji. It is wonderful to hear her voice and feel the Light. She says she will think of me on my birthday.

On February 4th, I am aware of her thinking of me and all of my interactions with people are sweet and calm.

In another cranial-sacral session, it is as if I am a baby emerging, being held by the heels in a lengthening stretch. I ask," Why was I born?" "Only to help – you don't need to do it all," Mataji says. It feels as though she and I are sisters. She has her arm around my shoulder, touching me, asking me to agree to help. Then I'm in the mountains, picking orchids for the altar. The air is clear. I am taking baby steps to the Divine. My lower back opens like a *cakra* but instead of lotuses, each *cakra* is an orchid. The light goes up my spine.

In the evening I walk to the Temple and see two full moons – one in the sky and the other a whimsical reflection caught in the Temple skylight. Everything feels special.

Spring 1993

How can L. and I develop a thread of trust? Her passing remarks or casual comments are meant to point out my mistakes. Why can't mistakes be taken as problems to be solved instead of judgements? Am I giving feedback as I promised myself I would? Or is it easier or more familiar for me to be critical in return? How can I address this?

Today I ask L. not to check me off her list in front of me; it makes me feel as though I'm just the next thing to do. Then I surprise both of us with the question, "Who is in charge?" We are supposed to be working together now – me as the program secretary, she as the backup. But she takes over and does everything. She says she only does what comes up and admits she feels jealous and pushed aside, especially because I do a good job with people. Her real interest is in expressing her creative side, she says, and her dream is to go to Mexico or South America. But she is starting to understand that unless she includes me and shows me what she knows I won't be able to do the work.

I'm hopeful, but as time passes I continue to be excluded from the flow of information on major areas such as finances, communication with Swami Radha and program planning. Some people have the big picture and some don't. That's okay, but as program secretary and Swami SP's right-hand assistant, what should I know?

I'm saying aloud my concerns, asking for the training, taking steps out of confusion, taking time for practice, time for myself. I bring forward suggestions but am stopped by an attitude of, "This is how it is," a resistance to change. I'm waiting it out, gradually earning respect, being consistent, being willing to be here for Swami Radha, being as clear as I can, thinking things through. Keeping it all in the Light.

I know Swami SP and L. are still reacting to my new position, but Mataji wants this change to happen. She asked me to learn everything about the Ashram and to help expand the vision. It is not my personal ambition. Maybe the changes will take ten or twenty years, but I have a feeling they will eventually happen. I am disappointed in myself for being up and down. I realize I do a disservice to myself if I let runaway thoughts interfere. I keep coming back to centre and it is okay.

How can the situation become cooperative instead of stressful? It feels as though something needs to shift but it's not up to me to make it happen. Please, Divine Mother, help me!

I remember my first boss at Alberta Ed saying that being criticized makes you think. The challenges of that job pulled me out from a housewife and daycare role to a professional consultant role. Here the criticism is bringing me to a higher standard in my office work, with more care toward details. And spiritually I am learning that instead of reacting to criticism, I can observe myself and practise surrender – learning to graciously accept whatever comes as an opportunity to break through old patterns. I'm also learning to take a stand when I need to, and to speak up when I do not agree with a direction.

In our meetings and day-to-day interactions, I am observing the other residents more closely – listening, asking questions, seeing their challenges and strengths, and understanding the dynamics of the group. I am extending beyond myself to ask: What is everyone else doing? How can I support them in their development?

This spring there are ideas stirring about a Radha Centre in Mexico. I haven't heard anything directly but I know from her stories that Mataji feels a strong connection to Mexico from the past and has always wanted to start something there. Recently some of her books were translated into Spanish and I think she is taking that as a sign.

In mid-May, Swami SP leaves for eastern Canada on a teaching tour. Mataji calls me to say I should report to her, not to Swami SP, about what is happening at the Ashram. Then she surprises us by arriving at the Ashram with plans to stay for a month. I am delighted to see her!

In our first meeting she says, "I have a delicate question to ask. I gave you the apartment so there would be space for the children, but now they are grown and living on their own. Would you like to move to Many Mansions?"

"Yes, I would love to!"

"Would the children understand?"

"Yes, of course," I say.

I love her. She keeps hugging me, saying she is glad I am here. I run off to start preparing.

My first day of being in Many Mansions feels as though I've entered another zone or atmosphere. I am tired from the shift but absolutely elated about being here. Everything is sorted out and in its place – downsized from a house to an apartment to a small room – and still I have what I need. I feel great gratitude to Mataji. The whole atmosphere of the Ashram has changed since she's arrived. And it's amazing to be living in her house, waking up here, doing practices, being able to talk to Julie about the teachings and my dreams each morning.

Swami Radha trusts me. I am tired and satisfied and nervous and very happy.

Mantra – again, hearing it before I start chanting. Where is it coming from? Aligning myself with the guru is very easy; chanting is very satisfying. Clarity of focus is the gift of being here.

I feel a wave of change, openness and support from Mataji. I feel as though I am finally learning what I am supposed to be learning. I want to know how she thinks about everything and everyone. She tells me about each person, their potential and obstacles, and encourages all of us to bring out the best in each other. Her observations range from details of day-to-day ashram life – living arrangements, the bookstore management, *Ascent* newsletter articles – to the responsibilities of initiation, the guru-disciple relationship and how *sanyas* blesses the family twenty-one generations before and after.

I watch her interactions with her other disciples. Mataji tells one woman that she still doesn't get it – that real knowledge means doing her own thinking, not memorizing the answers from a text. She challenges L. to work through her sickness. How can we change?

In the evenings I'm studying the Devi of Speech from the Kundalini book, preparing to teach a workshop in July. I plan to focus on the Divine Mother mantra and the influence of speech in our daily lives. I'm up early each morning, and before breakfast Julie and I discuss the Devi of Speech and do the exercises ourselves. This morning Mataji walks by and confirms our insights, saying to focus on the spark within, that the kingdom of God is within.

Time flies by. In the office we are getting ready for the summer courses. There is a kind of buzz sweeping over me as people come in and out. Everything starts to revolve around me and I have an idea that my work is to get things done, but is that right? I want to keep delegating, so we're all working together.

As the weeks pass I start to feel a growing anxiety about Swami SP's return. On Mataji's instructions I haven't been in contact with her and it feels as though a big shift has happened since she left. There is a different sense of openness and transparency in our approach. How will she react to it? I can't imagine going back to a limiting and hierarchical management style, but how will we go forward when she's here? She likes to keep things under her control and I'm sure she will be upset that we've made changes without notifying her.

Summer 1993

I'm at the office early this morning, doing bookkeeping. I take time off to gather some flowers for Swami SP's room to welcome her back. She comes into the office in an irate mood, unsettled, and demands to know what has been happening. I try to stay calm as I reassure her that the summer courses are organized and that the Ashram is fine.

I have no idea how everything is going to work out.

In the afternoon Mataji invites Swami SP to Many Mansions and asks me to serve tea in the garden screen house. I bring out the teacups and as I'm leaving Mataji invites me to join them. I sit quietly and listen as Swami SP describes her trip. She seems more cheerful and pleasant as she talks about the workshops and the students she has connected with on her tour. Mataji is very interested, wanting to hear about all the people she knows in Toronto and Ottawa.

Then she says, "Don't unpack your bags! Radha Centre Mexico is going to happen, and I'd like you to go down and find the place! You already have the experience of starting a Radha Centre and I know you've lived in another culture. I can't think of anyone better to take the lead there. How do you feel about that?"

Swami SP immediately responds that she is surprised but excited about the idea.

"Okay, then, start thinking about it. Get together with Don N and make arrangements as soon as you can. He can accompany you. We'll talk more about it later."

When she leaves my hands tremble as I clean up the teacups. Mataji comes over to me and says, "See? You don't have to worry anymore!" And she kisses me. I am full of wonder. Suddenly everything has changed, and with such finesse!

In the evening Mataji talks with me in a very helpful way. She says Swami SP is attracting her own disciples now, and she needs to establish something for herself from the ground up, shaping it in the way that suits her temperament and experience. Swami SP is aware of her past lives, she says, and has a bigger picture, so on that level she understands very well what is happening and why.

The day is full with people continually arriving for the summer courses. The world keeps moving in. I see Swami SP at supper and observe that she and Don N are so involved in leaving that their minds actually seem in Mexico already. Mataji is constantly here – caring, responding, wherever she is. She keeps her promise but she is not attached. She remembers. How to be focused and engaged and keep the promise and commitment to the Divine?

Tonight Mataji tells me that they will be ready to leave for Mexico by mid-August. They will scout for the new location and will return in mid-October. Then Swami SP will gather what she needs and move to Mexico to establish the centre and the society. L. is also leaving the Ashram for Mexico to learn Spanish in preparation for living at the Mexican Radha Centre.

This means that in six weeks I will be running the Ashram! Suddenly it is all happening so quickly!

Mataji says I can drive down on my day off to consult with her if I need help. She is leaving next week for Spokane, where she will be living in her new apartment. And it's only four hours away.

This evening Mataji and I are sitting together in the Sun Room. I feel that warm and vibrant feeling I remember so well from my first time here, when I asked her if I could call her Mataji. Tonight she invites me to use Many Mansions fully when she leaves. "Some people live at the Ashram and don't use what is here," she says. "Please use it; it is your birthright."

She asks who I would like to initiate me into *sanyas*, and says, "Taking *sanyas* is not necessary. It is only a gesture. Any swami can initiate another one. But you will have to initiate people into the mantra at some point, and the mantra initiation is the one that counts."

Then she gives me a gift of a lovely Japanese shrine, which just needs a little work. It is a wonderful treasure.

In my cranial-sacral session I see an image of myself in an orange shawl with Mataji. I am in a jungle and the shawl is my protection. I wrap it around me and I am like a flower.

Mataji is now in Spokane and I am feeling the loneliness of her absence. The house seems so big and empty without her. I do the Light in each of the rooms in the morning and night, filling the rice bowls each morning and night. I start sanding the Japanese shrine, preparing it for refinishing.

I lead the Devi of Speech workshop and it seems quite natural for me. The teachings come alive as people contact Divine Mother and see Her influence in their lives.

At lunch with Swami SP, she tells me she has written to Swami Radha saying that she feels she has fulfilled her duties as the Ashram's president and thinks she has done well. She wants to know what I will be doing at the Ashram. I tell her that in the next few weeks I would like to learn as much as I can from her – being with her in meetings, sitting in on the interviews that she has with the residents.

She says, "Some people have lived here for ten years and they already know the management and policies well enough to run the Ashram. You wouldn't need to."

I say, "Someone has to be responsible."

I keep bumping into this same resistance in Swami SP, even now as she is leaving. It feels as though she is trying to prevent me from doing what Mataji wants. What is behind it? Am I a threat to her? She seems suspicious of me, as if I have engineered her removal from the Ashram. But I was as surprised as she was by Mataji's proposal. All I know is that I love Mataji and want to surrender to her vision and do whatever I can to help the Ashram blossom. For two years I've offered help to Swami SP but it wasn't accepted. I could see that the Ashram would lose its vitality if it kept going down a narrow path, being controlled instead of opening to change.

The Ashram has a life of its own and we need to be receptive enough to follow it. I can envision our group working together, using each person's talents to the fullest. This is my hope. At the same time Swami SP is being offered a perfect opportunity to take her next steps toward the independence she is seeking.

Today I receive a note from Swami Radha:

> Dear Mary-Ann,
> I want you to know that you are indeed more on my mind than you may think. Swami SP will be in Mexico for a long time. You have to be the pillar in the Ashram, particularly from a spiritual point of view. Find out who can be of best assistance to you in the administration and how you can establish a good working relationship. Keep me informed of whatever news you have and let me know if there is anything else I can do for you. You are close. You have indeed a special place...
> Mataji.

Mid-August and we're celebrating the Ashram's thirtieth anniversary. At the guru *puja*, people prostrate before Swami SP. Some are her new disciples; the rest of us honour her office as president. I have the feeling that she is entangled here, attached to her position. Everything seems unclear about what will happen after she goes, even though she is leaving in a few days.

I'm thinking ahead and accepting the assignment of stepping forward. I have to give myself time to come into being. Everybody can step forward with me. My role is to encourage, direct, be there for people, delegate, get an overview, a bigger picture. Which way are we going? The Temple is for everyone; the Ashram is for everyone.

Mataji calls to tell me that she has asked Swami SP not to phone the Ashram under any circumstances while she is in Mexico. Am I breathing easier? "No one runs the Ashram except Divine Mother," she says. "Not me, not Swami SP, not you. Tune in."

Hearing her words reassures me and brings in awareness. I'm overjoyed by her voice. The Devi of Speech, the power of words. How do my words hold me back or help bring me forward to meet the challenge?

A wonderful day! I hear from the Spokane group that Swami SP is happy and relaxed and enjoying the weather in Mexico. At the Ashram the clouds have lifted. Everyone is relieved that we can talk freely to each other. In our management meeting we open up possibilities. How do we want to manage? What do we want to accomplish? We brainstorm and are receptive to ideas from all directions. We breathe a collective sigh of relief as we renew and step toward our potential.

I clarify my spiritual ideals for myself:

Be generous
Be clear
Be accepting
Be encouraging of myself and others
Offer more of myself
Have no fear
Ask questions

I am loving the Ashram, the beauty, the Light. The question slips in throughout the day, What would Mataji think or do in this situation? I am busy with people issues and too much to do, but I can watch my tone of voice and keep the connection.

I enter teaching, not plodding but soaring. The last course of the summer is Spiritualizing Your Life. Participants work in the morning and reflect and do practices together in the afternoon. Today we repeat the Divine Mother prayer and take a reflection from the Kundalini book. Gratitude is flowing from my body. I feel myself relax into Divine Mother. I feel wonder at Her sound and gratitude for the insights and challenges. I see the Light in the room and around people, and I am ecstatic to be back on track. I hear the words of the Divine Mother mantra resounding through the Temple, so many varied voices interwoven into one prayer, "May everything I do be taken as Thy worship."

During the next few weeks I receive confirming messages from people. My mother phones and says, "You were not a mother, wife or teacher. You were always an ashram lady. But how can you be running the Ashram if you're not a swami?"

One resident says, "It's as if Mataji is here. It's fluid."

Another says, "You wear the mantle with ease. Because you love this place and your work so much, it helps us."

Another resident asks a question. "You are not the president, you have not taken *sanyas*, you have only been here two years, yet you are still in charge, knowing very little about the Ashram. What does it mean to be the leader of the Ashram?" I say, "At the Ashram we do the guru's work. I surrender."

Mataji says, "I am in Mary-Ann's heart. She is in harmony with me. That is why it can work."

Fall 1993

September and the Ashram is quiet. Standing in the Mountain pose I'm thinking of the real me – moving inside, connecting. Become a reedlike thing available for the mantra. "What is behind the face?" Mataji asks. "Connect with that." I am not alone. I am not in charge.

I take time to absorb the supreme beauty of this place. My cells need that kind of nourishment. Today the residents have our own Spiritualizing Your Life class. We start by reflecting together, then everyone participates in work bees all over the Ashram. There is a sweetness as we gather together to do what needs to be done – picking apples, juicing apples, cleaning the Temple and harvesting the garden. I am in the Temple and we wash it until it sparkles. We are together in the work and in the way we work. I feel embraced by the colours, smells, tastes, softness, ease of relationships. Contentment.

At lunch all fifteen of us meet under the old apple trees outside of Main House and read our reflections to each other. It's a day where we come together as a whole, where we are all on the same level, doing our work with a feeling of joy. We accomplish so much in a short time. But the real accomplishment is the tremendous feeling of harmony, inclusiveness and unity we are building.

We gather for a visioning day. For the first time everyone sees where we are as an ashram and we ask where we want to go. We put up big sheets of paper on the wall, filling them with the range of work coming up and then with a list of our values. At the centre of the circle of values is our focus on Swami Radha's teachings and her message, "It is a privilege to serve those who seek the Most High." How can we work together and keep this ideal of selfless service alive? The meeting generates momentum. The action now is for each person to create a timeline for the work they are responsible for, and then we'll knit it all together. Our focus is "Do it now!" We want to respond quickly to whatever Swami Radha asks of us. We are taking the next step in our evolution, as individuals and as an ashram group.

I write to Mataji to express our commitment to her. "Dear Mataji: In the last years of your life, we want to do exactly what you want us to. Ask and we will do it. Anything to make your last years easier for you. We say yes."

We follow up with a planning meeting, where we can see the benefits of organizing our time. The changes and the results are evident. There is a transparency about responsibilities and communication. It is inspiring! It is also a testing time for me, with some people wondering what all the changes mean. There are a few silent critics. But as people bring their concerns forward there is a real sense of cooperation in an open, trusting way.

I take Mataji up on her offer and drive to Spokane to check in with her. She listens with interest to our new initiatives and encourages me not to stick to the old ways. She didn't. When she came back to Canada from India she had to adapt the teachings to the time and place. She expects the Ashram to expand with new vision. "Let it bloom," she says. "What do I have to do to prove that I am available and ready to support you?"

She advises me to learn the organization and administration of the Ashram, but more importantly to know the teachings and be able to teach anything. "And realize whatever the problems, they are a challenge that you must meet because the challenge is provided by the Divine. Remember that if I trust you and you trust my judgement, then you have to trust yourself. You can do it!"

Back at the Ashram, the office is in a state of chaos. Everything had to be moved to make way for the new photocopier. We completely empty the space, clean it and rearrange it. It looks new, different. Yes, things are changing – and not just physically. There are more people involved in the office work now – helpful, supportive people answering the phone, looking after guests, writing up the minutes, keeping track of *Ascent* subscriptions and doing the many office details. The guest registration is being switched to a computerized system, which will be much more efficient. There is an atmosphere of cooperation and support.

Mataji phones to say that Swami SP is in Spokane. She asks if my heart is beating fast. "Not to worry," she says, "I will take care of it." But my heart is beating fast. "When I was in your shoes I would have liked someone to talk to, but you have to learn to have faith in the Divine," she says.

Swami SP arrives and stays in her room all day. I phone her before dinner and we talk. She comes for dinner but doesn't look at me or say anything for the first five minutes. Then she criticizes the changes. I feel myself react. It's fast and we're back into the old dynamic. It won't happen again.

I go to my practices for support. Stillness comes with the breath. I feel a rocking all the way through my body, as if I am in Tara's arms again. How to approach Swami SP? Stay with the power of commitment rather than the power of criticism. I want to practise generosity and clarity.

This morning all of the managers meet with her. I can see that she is tired, sad and attached. At first she keeps referring to the lawyer as the real leader of the Ashram because he knows the legalities. Then she says that Swami Radha had asked her to be president and to head up the Ashram for a number of years. And now Mary-Ann is being asked to take the lead even though she is not the president.

This is the first time I've heard Swami SP acknowledge that I will be leading the Ashram, and I'm relieved to hear her say it.

She says that Swami Radha asked her to return the diamond ring, symbolic of the presidency, and that Swami Radha has taken back the official position of president again for now.

I tell Swami SP that it would be helpful if she could transfer the leadership to me in a more public way, so that others are clear. Right now the residents are uncertain about what is happening. She agrees and suggests a ritual in the Temple before she leaves for Mexico. I feel awkward about it but she assures me that we will do something nice. We eat lunch together and I can feel I've overcome my fear and am moving into a new place of trust in myself. I have trust in Swami Radha, who put me here. I feel as though I, too, am now accepting the position.

When we do the ritual in the Temple, Swami SP surprises me by expressing her delight and enthusiasm for what is happening at the Ashram. She calls me up to the front of the Temple and says, "Mary-Ann is one of the Divine Mother's finest handmaidens. You can turn to her if you need to have your antenna tuned." She passes me the Light and hugs me with an old warmth. I find it an incredible experience.

This morning she leaves for Mexico. I see her as a radiant Lakshmi. I know it takes a lot to turn negativity around, and she has done it. The spiritual side of her took hold and shone forth, and everyone relaxed with her. I hope the cooperation and goodwill in the Ashram are evident to her. She is off to make a fresh start and I think it must be exhilarating for her too. The location they discovered in Mexico is beautiful. The plan is definitely in effect.

I make another trip to Spokane to see Mataji. I feel and see her Light. This is where I ought to be. We sit down and immediately talk of the Ashram and the changes, and about the Radha Centres and people. Then she hands me a sparkly box. When I open it I see a ring with three diamonds. "This ring represents the first three *cakras*," she says, "and now we will see what happens! You can keep this one, but the presidential ring will be passed on and is not personal. It represents the lineage of teachers. When you become the president we will videotape the ceremony so everyone can see it. Eventually you will need to establish who the next president is and how she will be chosen." She makes it clear that the Ashram is not to be bound by men.

I drive back to the Ashram pondering what it will mean to become the president. It seems a bit much! What kind of commitment does it take to remember in this lifetime and others that I want to serve the Divine? I look at the three diamonds sparkling on my finger. The sparkles are within the diamonds. The outside is smooth and flat. Organization makes things smooth. What do I need? An advisory group connected to the Light to help with decision-making.

In November Mataji returns to the Ashram for an extended stay to support the transition. At our board meeting she comes in to talk to us about the presidency. She says it is essential that the president of the Ashram be a spiritual person. Administrative duties can be delegated to those who are skilled in that area, but having administrative ability should not be the deciding factor.

What is a spiritual person? I wonder. Was spirituality always a part of my life? Was it hidden? Does it mean that I could have accessed it earlier? How does it support me? What does it mean to say yes?

Winter 1993

It's a dark night in December, 3 a.m. Coziness of Mataji. Helping her up from bed, being with her. How sweet she is. An ongoing concern that she is in pain. She keeps faith in the Divine through the pain. Keeping on. "All saints eventually have illnesses to the weakest part of their system," she says.

"But when you live on faith, you accept what comes to you."

I am now working day and night. At night I sleep in Mataji's quarters in a very, very hot room, like an incubation process. I help with her needs and read to her when she wakes up. In the day I work with everything from petty cash to gearing up for Christmas.

She says to ask Swami Durgananda about initiating me into *sanyas*. I do, and we set my *sanyas* initiation date for February 2nd. The other night Mataji said it was the Ashram's karma to have me as president because I am not tainted by all of the past history and people's stories. She tells me that because I was available the Divine used me, not because I am the best yogi or the best teacher.

My inauguration into the presidency is at 3:30 p.m., December 30th, in the Temple. Mataji holds the ring and says the setting is designed to resemble a diamond in a lotus. I remember indications of the diamond lotus from a visualization in my Yoga Development Course more than ten years ago. I saw a diamond in the lotus in the pond outside Many Mansions and I knew it was for me. Today she leads us in a visualization of the diamond giving off Light. Everything is intense and quiet. She speaks of cooperation, communication and support. All the board members prostrate before her. She says we are a fine group of people – just what the Ashram deserves – and that I am someone on the path of Light.

After the ceremony I walk around the house, feeling like a bird hopping with no place to nest.

What has happened? I feel so ordinary to have such an extraordinary ring and legacy – one that I know requires devotion, stamina, strength of character. How does it happen, year after year, lifetime after lifetime?

I am unabashedly loving toward Mataji and feeling deep gratitude. My commitment is to offer this life to her teachings. I see even a tiny doubt prevents embracing her, so I focus constantly on my experience of her and the expression of the work that comes through her. It is a love beyond, behind, woven into her. My love is for her, for all she has carried, for what she has created, for how she has changed my life. She is the real helper, a bodhisattva.

The ring is heavy on my finger. I feel the weight of the legacy, my unconscious knowing, the effort of holding onto the Divine.

The Power Line

I'm trying to think of what my swami name could be, wanting something connected to Swami Radha. I suggest different options but they don't resonate. Standing in the kitchen Mataji asks me casually, "Why wouldn't you want 'Radhananda' as your name?"

"Does it matter that someone already used it?"

"Lots of swamis have had the same name. It's not a problem."

"Yes!"

Then she asks, "How would you feel about wearing blue instead of orange? It means changing from the Indian tradition. You would have to be strong enough to withstand the opposition. But blue is a more familiar spiritual colour in the West. People associate it with Mary's robes, with Divine Mother. You can also think of the blue of Krishna – as vast as the blue sky."

"Yes!"

I'm continuing my night vigils of responding and listening for
Mataji, helping her even as she helps me. Repeating silently,
I love you, you are Divine. I make up a little poem about our
special times together…

> I hear
> An echo your voice calls
> I awake from sleep
> and go towards the sound
> I come to help you up
> and you lift me to lightness in your embrace
> Later she walks trailing the fragrance of roses
> I sleep keeping an ear open for the call
> Again

Last night I slept just a few sporadic hours between calls.
My body feels porous with so little sleep. During the day I'm
very tired and am trying to clear my mind. I keep wondering
how I will do the teaching. We now have seventeen people
signed up for the YDC and so few experienced teachers.
What does this mean? When do I reach the point of saying
"no more," I need to recuperate? Is this the test? I've already
reached a point where I've gone beyond what I thought is
possible. How do I go on?

A few weeks into the YDC I can see that something has
taken hold and seems to be alive. Teaching Kundalini, the
adventure of self-discovery. A confirmation. I'm teaching
many of the courses with D. He has trouble listening to me.
The dynamic between us makes me question my perceptions.
Am I caught in a state of mind or is it actually happening? Is
he unable to tune into the flow between the student and me
without interrupting or reacting and taking control? When I
tell him my perceptions he says I am projecting, that he is just
a male symbol for me. I retract and find myself in the weird

position of protecting him from my comments.

I feel my perceptions are quite clear, but are they? Can I do it all – look after the Ashram, teach, look after Mataji at night? In between classes I'm in the office phoning and arranging guest visits, talking with the different residents. I chant, which I love, and go to satsang. It sustains me.

Tonight Mataji talks of how a pebble thrown into a pond creates waves going out in concentric circles. Each pebble does the same thing; it is not unique to any particular one. She seems to be describing the effects of the gurus and how they are all one in their purpose.

In the night she gets cross with me about my lack of awareness. "If you can't pick up something from the floor, how would you be able to pick up if someone is losing or taking energy?"

As D. and I continue teaching the tension builds between us. Today I am furious when he doesn't stick to our agreement. We said that it would be a summary day in class, where the students gather together their insights. But instead he keeps delving into the last paper until we are extremely overtime. When we teach we need to ask the questions; we don't need to get involved in drawing out the answers. I am also concerned about keeping Mataji waiting for me, knowing that I have the whole night ahead of me.

In the evening she seems irritated with me. I do nothing right, from using her paper and pen to tucking her in wrongly. How will I become Radhananda? I let go any defensiveness. Surrender to what is. She goes back to sleep, and when she wakes up she is gentle. She says I will be president for years to come and suggests I make a pamphlet on initiation. I remember back to the feeling of my mantra initiation – bowing to the gurus and the altar, being beside her and her small table with the almonds, rose petals, powders and water, my mala around Tara, Mataji's whispers to me to do everything she says, that she will tell me.

Guru is the focus. Crabby night or expansive night – can I keep my focus on her? Sleepy night or bright night – can I keep my focus on her? Guru as the point of love; doing it for love. What would I sacrifice? When I massage her feet I don't know how to do massage, but I say over and over, "I love you. You are the Divine." The fingers find a way and there is a connection between us. Doing something for her, not for myself. Bring in the focus, bring in the love, bring in the action.

She is in pain. What does she need? My mind focuses, attentive to her. Her trust gives me the trust to trust myself. What if my work is to keep myself in shape, mentally, physically, spiritually for the work with her? No task is too hard.

In preparation for my *sanyas* initiation Mataji asks me to reflect on commitment and sacrifice.

Commitment – I need to keep the commitment to myself and the part that knows. Commitment to the work, to Swami Radha, all else fades away. She is not an image in the sense of a beautiful appearance, but an image of what it looks like to be dedicated to the teachings and what this way of life means.

When I look back at my life I see that attachments fell away or I was gently tugged away from them. My mind sees the pull, then it lets go. But was there a sacrifice? The ring – the way it sits on my finger – what is the commitment I am taking on? It's like a gateway shuts off part of the world and I step through. It happens at each point of transition or evolution, from being a teacher in the school system to a manager consulting teachers, to teaching in this expansive way.

A raven flies by the window, wings outstretched, sun gleaming on wingspan.

Did I ever want those other things anyway?

My initiation is tomorrow. I spend the day in my room sorting through the clothes I will give away. I chant for everyone I know. Then I listen to the recording of what she said to me at my inauguration and I study the eighteenth chapter of the Gita on renunciation. I try on the blue silk sari. It's beautiful, like a waterfall.

February 2nd. The initiation ceremony is in the Temple early in the morning. I bow to the pictures of Swami Radha and Gurudev. Sitting on the tiger skin with Swami Durgananda and surrounded by a circle of the other swamis, we chant. I light the candle between the two gurus. In the silence that follows I receive the *brahmacharya* and *sanyas* mantras from Swami Durgananda.

When the ceremony is complete, I go to Mataji and bow before her and she touches my head in blessing. I walk to the lake, my blue sari flying in the wind, and throw in the tuft of my hair saying, "I throw away the part that thinks it can't. I CAN!"

Swami Radhananda – new life, new person.

I go to the Temple and do the Divine Light at each of the seven windows. When I come back to Many Mansions, Swami Radha greets me with three white snow roses from her winter garden – symbolic, she says, for being able to bloom in the cold.

She has a look of supreme delight and a sparkle in her eyes. "I think the work will succeed," she says. "You are the one designated to carry on. Many people do not think deeply enough to understand the teachings. Someone is designated, even if they don't know it. You are 'it.' Others will come to you."

I will try my best to be Radha, the love of Krishna, to

hear the flute, to hear the messages without clouding my vision by emotions, needs or desires. I want to hear Swami Radha and do what she asks and love her no matter what. Beyond matter.

She asks me to think deeply about each line of the Divine Light mantra. The Divine Light Invocation itself is an initiation, she says. She added the last line because she thought if she understood even a little, she would always want to grow into Light. Put all your emotions into that thought, "I am ever growing into Divine Light."

My first night as a swami is one of the worst. Mataji yells at me about a pair of pants I can't find, asks me if I hear her neck crack when I lift her hips. "You need more awareness in listening!" I get the pills confused and lie that I had written it down. She makes a huge sign – "Please use awareness with my medication" – and puts it on her desk so I will remember.

A day of tiredness and of learning my new name, "Swami Radhananda." It is hard to see myself as that name, almost an embarrassment of how precious it is, how special. I feel badly all day about how I disappointed Mataji last night, and sad about how sick she is. She is so weak that she can barely move and the doctor has come to see her. "Renounce the worlds" seems supremely important.

Over the next week the snow roses continue to bloom on my altar. I really like my robe. It feels so wonderful. Sometimes I feel extremely giddy with so much Light and I'm trying to figure out why I would need more mantras. Other times I feel absolutely exhausted – so little sleep, no time to think. Time is going too quickly. I'm trying to hold on physically. It feels like so much responsibility – teaching and more teaching, trying to keep my eyes open at odd hours of the night to read to Mataji.

Tonight she gives me some advice to pass onto the young women about life and sex. Ask them what their relationship is based on. How many lifetimes have they been a mother for their own emotional needs? Get the facts – what is love, what is sex? How do they bring in quality and consideration? Not many men can love – they tire of their sexual partner and look for younger women. Don't have romantic expectations that may not be met. The only real love is the Divine.

She talks to me about initiations. "When you initiate someone," she says, "ask them to give you their greatest attachment. You will be able to tell from their papers. It is not necessarily money. Who would you initiate? Remember someone did it for you."

I am disoriented by lack of sleep.

It's the end of February. I've been on nights since early December and today Mataji says, "You will be doing service in this office for many years. You must look after your body because people's needs and desires and emotions will erode your central nervous system." She says we need quality time together and she is taking me off night duty. Now I will just be with her in the evenings. It's a relief.

Mataji asks me to sit at the front of the Temple in every satsang. It's a challenge to sit up there! I feel like a child. She trains me by having me sit on a chair beside her whenever she leads satsang. She asks me not to fidget or to be concerned about where and how people are sitting. Sit still. It is my chance to practise being "up front" while she is here – a challenge to the part of me that just wants to blend in or disappear.

I've been a swami for just a month now and I am astonished when Mataji says I should initiate Bruce, a young man who has been on the YDC and has terminal cancer.

She says he could choose to die at the Ashram if he wishes. "Initiating him," she says, "will be like holding the hand of a dying person or being with a sick person in pain. It is the same." I should put his first and last papers from the course in my altar, and then once a month, forever, include him in my prayers. She says to ask Divine Mother what I am to do. Bruce should do the Light ten times a day and reflect on each line.

I think of the intimacy of an initiation with him and what it means.

I've been too long in the minds of seventeen other people, eight straight days on the YDC, teaching. I can't reflect for myself anymore. I've forgotten how. There is so much work to do. I can't sort out my job. President, program secretary, teacher, swami. It's complicated. I just feel tired. And I'm sad to see Mataji continuing in so much pain. What can we do for her?

O Divine Mother, sacrifices, sacred acts, offerings.... How will the work succeed if I keep it limited within my range? It has to be spiritual and administrative – not one or the other. I chose this name. Now live up to it.

At lunch Mataji asks how I am. I say, "Sad and tired." She tells me there is nothing wrong with me, that she had the same experience when she started. When I am in intense activity with others I need to protect myself and keep myself filled with Light. She gives the advice that Gurudev gave to her. In emotional interactions keep my arms crossed to protect the solar plexus and my ankles crossed to retain energy. But this alone isn't enough. She says to keep my emotions steady and don't allow other people's emotions to ignite mine. Keep interactions at a distance as if they are outside myself, almost like a business conversation. Don't be drawn in. There is an exchange of energy with all beings at all times. Can I be aware of where my energy is going or what I am taking from others?

I tell her that focusing on the rings is also an instant reminder of the Light, a reminder of the help that is available.

Spring 1994

Tonight I take the president's ring to bed and hold it in my hand during sleep. I wake up at 3:30 a.m. with the ring still in my hand and a sense of expectancy. I have asked for a dream about the presidency.

In my dream I am at the power line, seeing the poles and lines going far back into the distance.

I reflect on the symbol "power line." Power needs a line. There is a line of power that the electricity passes through. People can use the power how they will. The power comes from a generator – generations of people connected through sacred power, sacred trust. Being aligned with a power – the power of the mantra, the power of conviction, of commitment, of truth. It's a force that is needed for the work. For something to work it has to be connected to the power line – the line of gurus, the lineage of Saraswati. The power line starts at the source, and the power is received all along the way. It is a connecting place. The power is received and runs through it.

My first interpretation of the dream is that the unconscious has spoken and confirmed my connection to this lineage. The work needs a line to flow through and I am there.

What is happening? Make use of the time with Mataji. She only had six months with her guru. She will be leaving the Ashram soon to return to Spokane.

Again this evening she gives me teachings about sex. She says to be emphatic about asking women to look at the facts. She says that men are sexually attracted to many women and propagate for pleasure. Women should be aware of the rhythms of their own body and its fertility cycles, and not romanticize love and confuse it with sex. For centuries women have been considered property, to be handed over undamaged at marriage. Now it's important for women to establish their financial independence and break that dependency on men. She advises building a friendship first instead of seeking acceptance. She has seen that some women will turn to other women for the experience of closeness.

Mataji says if her disciples don't recognize her in the teachings, what is the point? It is not about her body. She asks me how I teach and about how my mind works. I tell her about my reflections on Divine Mother in the Temple, how I speak to Her and She responds. She says I'm too concrete. I need to read more texts and think more subtly.

Tonight she gives an inspiring talk in the Temple on Divine Mother. She reads her poem about a white bird arising out of the darkness of her mind. She asks the bird to fly to Divine Mother to receive a message, then come back and tell her. After the reading there is silence. I experience my own visualization of a bird flying to Tara to receive her message for me. Something happened in the silence that my mind could have described in terms of Light or vibration. I chose to put it into a form that I could relate to, although it wasn't actually a form. It was something else that needed words.

At the end of satsang one of the women came up and prostrated first before Swami Radha, then me. I felt so awkward! Swami Radha tells me that if people *pranam* to me, I should touch them on the back of the head and say, *Om*

Namah Sivaya. It is not personal. Let the Light flow through and give the blessing.

Bruce's initiation is on my mind. I ask her more about it. I am still not quite ready. She says he should prepare by repeating the Divine Mother prayer and reading the guru and disciple book[1]. The initiation will not be a complete one, she says, but more of a gift for a good start in his next life. She mentions the power line dream as an indication of what is available to me. I know I have her guidance and support and I am willing to give back from that place of Light, to keep him in the Light, and to encourage what he has to learn.

I have another intense conversation with Mataji. She says the temptation for me in my position would not be money, fame or relationship. The temptation would be to leave because people can't hear the teachings. "Remember it may not be their time," she says, "or their karma." I ask her how she stays fresh. She says to be in the Light, to move in the Light, and to talk as if to a new group of students. Ask them to answer their own questions to awaken their intelligence. Challenge them to think deeply for themselves.

"A charismatic leader is not what is needed," she says. "The Ashram needs someone who is practical and willing to learn." She has observed that some of her disciples over the years have been given initiations, positions and even jewelry to remind them of how precious they are, and yet they remain depressed, jealous, unbelieving or unhappy. They have a choice and don't take it.

I am Radhananda and that means it is possible to connect.

---

1   *Guru and Disciple* was a pamphlet published by the Ashram in 1959. Portions of it now can be found in *In the Company of the Wise* and *On Sanyas* by Swami Sivananda Radha.

She tells me to be patient with people. Everyone does not understand or develop at the same time. Trust the Divine. Everything is change. As I change so will my perspective. But people need time to bring about their changes.

She looks at me and asks, "Even if no one trusts you, will you still do the work? Can you trust the Divine through all the changes and situations?

"Do what is most challenging," she says. "Delegate what you already know so that other people can learn. Expand into new areas. Have many heads, like the goddesses. Don't allow yourself excuses. The main thing is to ask the Divine to blow away the clouds from your mind. Face the mind and not all the clutter that surrounds it. Take time to study, reflect and practise.

"Don't push, which is your tendency. The flower will grow and develop on its own. Even if there is something another person isn't doing, you don't need to reject him or her. For example, you may not do accounting well but it doesn't mean you won't do anything else well or learn. Think of people as an orchestra. Each plays a different instrument, which doesn't necessarily create the sound you like."

Talking to her is like turning on the Light of understanding. I need to refocus on the real work and not get confused about what is important. Everyone can learn.

The YDC is over. "Have a celebration," Mataji says, "with treats for the students and for the residents! Enjoy the victories!"

Happiness that as a group we can come together in fun, just as we can come together in commitment, and we can come together in the Light of the Temple, simple and beautiful. Everything seems right. Together we are many-headed, many-armed.

In the planning meetings we come together with cooperation – cooperating with our sense of responsibility and our willingness to do what needs to be done. Our talk at the meetings isn't just about what we do. It is also about how we are, how we relate to each other, and what is happening in the moment of being together.

Something comes together in myself too, as I listen to my body in a yoga pose, or as I listen to students in class. Attention, waiting, listening and listening until something else comes in. Last night, I was planning the Kundalini course – working with my own reflections, working from the practices, waiting for the moment of understanding. It comes.

I feel strongly her sacred trust in me.

Mataji has a soft, gentle look, and she seems so well. Why do the eyes have such power? "You can close your eyes and go inside," she says, "to break up the energy drain."

I am leading the residents in a Kundalini Overview workshop. Tonight the men talk about how they look at women, sex and gratification. What a shock! These people, who I thought I knew, are transformed. I am suddenly aware of men and power and how it manifests. Their talk of women as objects and of how they do not honour women is quite incredible. When the men get together there is a force that seems loud and different. Can they allow themselves to soften and honour the feminine? How can I bring the women together? What would that look like? What is our work?

The Kundalini system is certainly effective. It reveals everything – where we really are, the obstacles and the potential.

At supper Mataji talks about how we are created by the Light for a purpose. The Light creates us. Do we really think we create ourselves through sex? About teaching, she advises, "Don't enter the psyche of another with your insight. Keep it to yourself. Just ask the questions and observe what comes back."

Our resident Kundalini workshop ends and Mataji says she is so pleased with the course. Where did I get the idea of reflecting on the symbols and the mantras? I said from her – from the Path of Liberation workshop I did in 1980! She said reflection helps people to understand, but they don't understand Kundalini until they've experienced it.

A bubbling day filled with Light and high feeling.

She is very happy about the cooperative work here and how everyone is being trained in Kundalini. "And you must have good karma," she says, "to come into a ready-made ashram."

Before she leaves to return to Spokane, I tell her that the presidential diamond ring had been causing a reaction on my finger. She exchanges it for a ring she calls "the pearl of great price." The pearl is huge and reminds me of the temple. But does this mean I'm not meant to be the president?

The end of May and it's my first trip outside the Ashram to teach workshops. I start at 6:30 a.m., driving to Calgary. I'll stay overnight at the Radha Centre, then fly to Ottawa and Toronto to teach.

Driving alone, I have time to think. The mountains in the misty distance holding up the sky remind me of the great teachers in the background, holding up seekers. I'm trying to make my everyday life spiritual as Mataji does. I see that other people are willing too. How to keep perspective without being drawn in?

Mountain air streams through the windows and lodgepole pines flash by. I'm alone, with everyone in my head. How does it become so intimate? I think of two of the ashram men and their competition with each other. They love the same guru, how can they not love each other? Why don't they want to get to know each other better?

Into Alberta where the mountains are huge, sometimes hidden, then suddenly appearing, grouped, but each with its own rounded or peaked face. I stop at Storm Mountain for lunch. The mountains are so close. Driving on, past the great continental divide, yet there is no division – just one space and an imaginary line. Entering the city of Calgary, everything speeds up, lanes of traffic, masses of housing tracts on hillsides.

Sweetness seems to flow along with me, carrying me here and filling me up, waves of Light and mantra.

Calgary Radha Centre has a new arrangement of teachers and residents. How far do I go to support their growth and direction? My responsibility is to speak to what I see but everyone has to take responsibility for their own life and evolution. Being outside the Ashram I see myself new and observe the leap of the last three months.

At the Radha Centre in Ottawa the students are familiar to me and the teachings are alive and well. It is wonderful to be here. We enter the Kundalini system in the new way – looking at the *cakras* and reflecting on the mantras. The director is excited about the approach and we have good talks in the evenings as we walk along the canal – beside fields of tulips, to the Parliament Buildings, and into the National Gallery.

The group seems to get so much out of the workshop. The work they have already done on themselves is obvious, and the workshop gives them the opportunity to go further. It is remarkable to see the way the Kundalini system leads them to their next step.

At the workshop outside Toronto the group is new and tentative – afraid of what the process will bring. I go gently.

Each evening there is more resistance and tentativeness. I start thinking that I need to explain everything but realize that's not it. They can only take in a little, so I end early.

In Toronto I stay with a former ashram resident, an old friend. She is here working and living alone to strengthen herself. Entering her small apartment I can feel the effects of her focus on spiritual practice. I notice my picture on the altar beside Gurudev and Mataji. Strange. What is this? Who am I? I tell her that I don't need to present myself as a teacher or guru. It's not the time. I may be in training for it, but that is a difficult idea for me to hold in my mind right now. I can do the day-to-day work fine but how do I become this other? We continue to talk into the evening and night – on *sanyas*, on taking the next step and living through it.

After the last few days I just want simplicity. When she goes to work I go for a walk, do some Hatha, visualize Light, repeat the Divine Mother prayer and feel better.

In the workshops over the weekend, there are women who have serious needs with family illnesses, a friend who committed suicide, and other tragedies. I feel that something is carried with me from the Ashram, and it reaches out and touches them.

Each night we come home to the altar and settle into the noisy city sounds. I transform the noise into a prayer to Divine Mother. Where is She in me? The sweetness that seems to flow from the Ashram is all around me. I am thinking about the ashram group, about my involvement, my promise, my duty. It is like seeing myself from outside myself.

Images and thoughts of the day come through. It feels as though the Temple and my practices become part of the courses – the sounds of mantra, the feel of the mala beads. I hear the prayer as a whisper through the city sounds and I talk to Divine Mother and think of Her space within me. She is the Radhananda part. She grants me understanding as I learn. It is almost as if the city noise itself becomes the sweetness from the Ashram and connects me to the "She" in me. How to honour Her?

Walking through Toronto in a sari, people hardly notice. Workshops, meetings with friends of the Ashram, shopping, in-depth talks with my friend, then the taxi comes to take me to the airport. I fly back to Calgary and drive home.

Entering the Temple again – beauty, calm, a heavenly sense. Being present in the company of the Light. Feeling space, treasure, preciousness, welcoming vibrations. The fragrance of the irises comes right into me. Has the sun brought the fragrance to life? Or do I allow it in by opening myself?

I am reminded of the workshops and how Divine Mother appeared after we called Her name. I recognized her preciousness in glimpses – Oh, there She is! Oh, this is a gift from Divine Mother! I thank Her for what was given. She is surprisingly available – through the sense of smell, taste, sight, hearing, touch. Focus on Her and there She is! Even in words and tones of voice. The sweetness that was carrying me – it came from the Ashram and it came from Her.

I feel gratitude for the reality check. Divine Mother is everywhere.

Summer 1994

The time seems right and I prepare for the ceremony with Bruce. Awake in the night, I wonder what it means and exactly how we should do it. Then early in the morning I get ready and set up on the beach. I see it as a ceremony designed to make him aware of the choices he has. The ceremony can plant a seed. I feel joyful and am brought very consciously to the present moment.

I tell him that all are precious in the eyes of Divine Mother. Initiation means the start of something and to make space in his life for the Light and Divine Mother. Pray and fervently make it real. I see that Bruce wants to do this and it is his victory.

During the ceremony I feel a bee buzzing near me as if I were a flower. It comes near my mouth, then to Tara, then to Bruce. After the ceremony Bruce looks at me with open love. The next day he asks if I am his guru. I say that I am his witness. It is his commitment I have witnessed.

A few days later he is in the hospital. His family decides to take him back east to their home. Before he goes he returns to the Ashram and we all gather together in the Temple to pray for him and pass a candle with our prayers. The chandeliers become very bright as lightning flashes along the lake and thunder roars.

I am starting to understand that my responsibility as spiritual director of the Ashram is to act on intuition, to care for and to bring out the best in others and myself. My commitment is based on loving Swami Radha, being concerned and helping. My position demands growth and change and responsibility. I have to be willing to learn from others and to show all sides of myself. Something else runs the Ashram. My place is to be a handmaiden, a willing worker.

We are also learning together as a group. In the ashram board meeting today, I ask the hard questions, not allowing undercurrents. We have to learn not to repeat the mistakes of other management groups or think ourselves immune. After our meeting, I think I have never been braver in my life.

As we prepare for the summer workshops and influx of students, I notice that one of the young swami women, Swami PR, is obviously attracted to a student. Sexuality? Love? What is my duty? What ought I to do? The question rests in my mind. I will bring it forward to Mataji on my upcoming visit.

I drive to Spokane. The plan is to stay here and look after Mataji while Julie goes to the Ashram to teach a Hidden Language workshop on the Triangle pose. But when I see Swami Radha she looks so peaked and little and weak that I am afraid she won't have long to live. I'm not familiar enough with how to help her fragile body. She is in too much pain and I do not want to create more. It is so sad to see her in pain again. If I stay here, all I can do is make it worse. Julie should stay and look after her. I have to do something else.

We are on her veranda together and I say, "I will do anything. I see there is no way I can help you physically, but there is another way I can help. I will look after you through the work. This is the best I can do." I don't know whether I say it out loud. I just know that at this moment I have a feeling of love, of my heart opening and opening and something entering in. And I know that I have to do what I have to do. Something happens... I can never understand these things... this overwhelming sense of love. I love her and my commitment at this point is so deep.

There is a promise made between us. "I'm going back.... I'm going back to teach." It's like an echo from the past, words that have been spoken before.

I have a strong, strong feeling, a deep heartfelt connection. It doesn't have anything to do with her body or my body. I have this knowledge that I am "it" and that I have a big job ahead. The job now is to go back and teach. I have to do it now. It is decided.

When I get back to the Ashram she is with me. She is not her body. I start the Triangle workshop and do the reflections. I connect with the dream I had when I was with her in Vancouver, where she turned into a white triangle and transformed back into herself when the triangle was put in water. The teachings are so powerful that they will always connect back to her, and she will be here. We keep repeating the Triangle in class, keeping the focus.

I have an experience when I am in the pose, where I am encased in a pyramid shape filled with Light, seeing the heart *cakra* triangles within me. Swami Radha is before me and we are both inside the triangle. We are looking at each other with love. Shouldn't she be resting? But she loves the Light. Then I am in the Temple and the Temple becomes a brilliant circle within a pyramid. My hands are filled with Light. My palms are radiating and streaming out Light.

The workshop is very powerful. Days later I still have the feeling of the triangles within me like tattoos of Light.

I am a vessel – that is the feeling for me. I am her vessel. This feeling generates commitment. Not just "I am committed to the work," but a promise and a knowing that there is no other way I can be. She I am. And from this perspective I know I have to detach from the details of the Ashram and focus on what is important.

A quiet moment. Feeding the fish in the pond. They know about feeding time and are ready to approach the person who feeds them. The Ashram is the place of teachings. Readiness, willingness. All the people who come here are ready to be fed on many levels. We are ready for the summer and a whole new approach. Approaching the goddess.

Some days I feel paper-thin, as if my skin is transparent and people can see right into me and I can see into them.

I remember the water from satsang last night coming on to my head in drops, and I felt as though I was on the banks of the Ganges – sun, large expanse of water, beads of water dripping from me, this same feeling of drinking in the mantra as we chant – drinking it in, using the mantra to bring the fullness of life and purpose.

It doesn't matter if I'm here at the Ashram or there with Mataji, just be in her heart. I am practising saying what needs to be said, not afraid of being disliked or misunderstood. Putting this into action. The teachings are worth more than anything else.

My job is to teach the Light and to be the custodian of the teachings. Everything else is irrelevant. Everyone has a place here. The challenges come. My prayer is to be porous enough to absorb the Light and teachings, strong and straight enough to put them into effect. I am willing to make mistakes. Even mistakes can be an offering, if reflected on and learned from.

One area I'm working on is developing my understanding of men. I often react quickly and impatiently to them. I want them to change. I need a different mindset but it means going slowly to build relationships on trust. I don't want to be their mother. If anything, I want to be a liberator so they are free. But I also want to expand my own awareness so that I am free. It will be a process of trust, discrimination and learning.

I continue to observe what is happening between Swami PR and the woman she is attracted to, wondering how to approach. The relationship seems to be deepening. When I report back to Mataji she says the student should go, Swami PR should stay. Her *gurubhais* are her true friends.

When I meet with Swami PR, she tells me how embarrassed she was to talk about her relationship. She felt trapped in attraction. Now it's a test of the support and grace that the Ashram can offer her. She could gain strength through a *tapas*. She says she is willing to do the work, whatever it takes.

I dream that a situation arises where I have to make

people accountable for their actions. It is the part of my job that I don't like but is essential.

Summer – people, courses, teaching. The people in the courses look different, finer, when they leave, as if they have been through a process of refinement, adjustment, alignment – like diamonds forming under pressure, being polished to an intensity and sparkle.

I am at this place of new learning of not being involved in all the details, turning that level over to others. I am focusing on my Radha nature.

Going Through the Fire

Fall 1994

Our visioning and planning meetings are even more directed this fall. Now when we plan ahead for the year we know what we can do. I know what I can do. My time with Mataji of working night and day makes my ashram day shift seem like half-time.

My summer visit with Mataji brought forward an intense desire to do, because she looked so frail and thin and in need of support. I came back to the Ashram with an intense desire to help her. This fall, after I visit her, I feel an intense desire to change myself, to place myself in the fire, to go beyond myself in order to live my purpose. Sometimes it seems impossible and sometimes it just slips in, as if it has to be there for the benefit of something greater than me. Impatience is one of my traits. It has only been a year, no need to be impatient. Be patient with myself. Be patient with others. There are steps to wholeness. How long does the seed wait?

Gurudev told Mataji that her whole life was a preparation for the teachings and the work she had to do. All of us are prepared – ready or not! What am I prepared for? Letting go of who I am? I am willing to prepare but I can't make it happen. What is it that happens? There is the ongoing work, people, emotions. I'm prepared to move forward, but what else does it take? Not getting stuck. Preparing to be in a different state or to take a different stand.

In the statue on my altar, Krishna supports Radha and Radha supports Krishna. "Without you," He says, "I am nothing." At the Ashram people are supporting what is best for their spiritual development. I am supporting Swami Radha's work, what she has set in motion. One of my goals is to be transparent, to harbour no secrets. I will talk to anyone about any situation.

One thing I can see is that I have to learn to work and live with men in intimate settings and relationships – *gurubhais* and initiates. I don't have to withstand the kind of criticism Mataji went through, but I do have to establish and test myself by working with the men who are here, and then transferring that knowledge to understand the other men I meet in classes and workshops.

Divine Mother has the plan, and it is perfect.

Mataji says when I first applied to live at the Ashram it couldn't happen. It wasn't because she didn't want me but because I had to gain life experience. Then after a number of years I had everything I needed. But I was so focused on the Divine and my desire to be at the Ashram that I never paid enough attention to the money. She was concerned. Would I make it? Why was it taking so long? Finally she asked me how much money I had, and like a child, I told her. Would I think she wanted the money? She said she had to take the chance. She risked not being liked. She risks constantly.

I, too, am risking not being liked. I'm putting the ideals and ethics of the Ashram first. Mataji knows I am at the beginning, still young and inexperienced in my position. But she knows I am rooted in the teachings and can be her instrument. She says when I make mistakes to tell her.

There are times when I don't know. In the situation with Swami PR, who is still attracted to her absent friend, it is not the individual but the situation that has me not knowing. I don't know what to say, or what Mataji wants, or how to approach. I have a feeling I'm stepping out onto a limb. I am on edge, on the edge. I keep Mataji informed at each phase, asking her what I should do. I keep the other residents informed.

When I report to Mataji, she points out that I need to become more sensitive to each situation. I didn't take enough time to reflect about how Swami PR would feel if I brought up her attraction in the resident group. It is new for her, unexpected, unplanned. Was I being too demanding, exposing her situation to the larger group? I don't want to justify my mistakes. I want to surrender and learn to think through the situation as deeply as I can.

If Swami PR drops *sanyas* and leaves, would I be responsible? Mataji says that there are many reasons why people behave the way they do. It takes time to find out. Each person's commitment to their spiritual life is also based on their karma. She says the hardest thing for me to do is to let people leave, but sometimes the Ashram is not the best place for them. And sex is a powerful force.

I am overcoming any hesitancy to tell Mataji what is happening in the moment. I'm going beyond my likes and dislikes, going beyond my pride or thinking I know when I don't. My victory is to use the work I've been given to make changes in myself. I am doing the best I can with sincerity and devotion.

Swami PR sits in our resident group tonight, refusing to talk about anything. She is laid back in her chair, looking at everyone else, writing loudly. When she is asked to participate she protests, "Is this a confessional?" Her anger enters with a vengeance. Later one of the residents challenges me on how I am handling the situation. Maybe I shouldn't be here.

After the group I step out into the night, following the moonlit path around the garden and seeing the growth, hearing the quietness. I follow the path down to the beach, saying the mantra as I walk. The mountains flash as if they have lightning behind them and the negative looks positive. The world is translucent.

I take the pearl ring to bed, holding it through the night, and wake up with the thought, Don't say anything. Mataji sends a message for me not to work so hard at saving people but to save myself for the important work later.

I leave to go on a teaching tour for a few weeks. When I get back I become very ill with what is diagnosed as shingles. The rash flares up and is painful. System overload. Too much travel, teaching, talking, being projected upon. I'm trying to figure out who I am. It has been a time of turmoil. What is my job? This is the question I keep coming back to. Swami Radha phones and says, "Everyone comes to you. You can't take it all on. You have to depend more on the Divine."

I hear that Swami Radha is in pain and we chant for her in the Temple. I am sad and feel unready. Would I have enough understanding now to carry out her wishes if she dies?

Julie calls from Spokane to say that Swami M. is leaving the work. I have known him for more than fifteen years and he has been Swami Radha's disciple for even longer. He has decided that the vow of *sanyas*, renouncing the world, is too much and he wants to leave his commitment. He doesn't seem concerned that Swami Radha is in pain, and that his leaving now will add to her pain. He comes back to the

Ashram to tell the residents his decision and to be disrobed by the swamis. He seems arrogant and does not say thank you in any way. What would it take to crack that shell of pride? After he is disrobed we suggest he leave immediately as the situation is disturbing for everyone.

Many of the residents are in an emotional state. I am trying to stay calm, relaxed and let Krishna sort it all out. Someone else will have to go to Spokane to help out, and we will work within the limitations. The Ashram expands and contracts; we surrender to the flow.

I think of commitment. As a mother commitment meant looking after the children and daily caring. Commitment is not glamorous; it is just being there. I think of Swami Radha being committed to people for twenty years or more, and how they just walk away with the teachings and all of her efforts. Where do they go? Her commitment shines as she starts again, through all the disappointments. Commitment is never giving up on the Light in each person. Maybe the commitment is not to the person but to the Light. She keeps telling me to trust the Divine.

Separation. How could I ever separate from my heart? I put her there by constant focus and love. She is part of me. Separate from her blessings? She and I have made a promise. She gave me a thread that connects us forever. I have seen the looks of love that shine from her eyes in blessings. Sometimes her voice comes through me clearly. She is my spiritual mother who has imbued each cell with Light, who is the flame in my heart.

I pull the group together and we gather at Main House to make Christmas cookies, dispelling the idea that commitment is hard. We can do it joyfully. There are many options and possibilities. I see that no one is indispensable.

I feel proud of our ability to regroup. I am glad that we can keep our connection and our heritage and expansiveness, that we can know each other well and still work together and encourage one another and change.

I'm alone studying when Swami PR comes into the room. I ask her what is happening. We start out informally, but I keep asking what is happening. She says that talking things through doesn't work for her and she knows she can't do it alone. She has no trust.

I ask, "What would help you? Can you work in the group? Do you want to be by yourself? I haven't seen you for two days."

She yells, "You're wrong! I was in the house yesterday – it's only been one day!"

Whatever I say she yells back. With the illness it's as if I have no buffer for my emotions – it is peeled away. I leave the room and cry and cry.

I call Mataji and she says to let her go. Swami PR decides to take a leave of absence. I feel as though I have been going through the fire with someone, holding on, not knowing what will happen, learning to trust the situation, learning to trust the Divine.

Swami Radha phones again to say that one of the other residents had called to talk with her about moving from the Ashram to live on her own and gain skills. She blasts me for expecting too much of this woman. She says I need to think things through. Why would I ask anyone to leave before I found a replacement? I'm going too fast. She also tells me that Julie is not in a good space and she is planning to send her to Vancouver. I feel exhausted.

What is the power and the stretch of surrender? What does it feel like? Sometimes surrender is the glorious feeling of bowing down to her that I like so much. Sometimes it is a pull into an unknown area where things don't make sense.

I want to ask her how to make a decision when there is no intuitive message from the Divine. When I can't tap into any insight all I can do is trust her, love her.

An internal shift seems to be accompanying my physical illness and recovery. I'm finding new ways to do things. I feel raw and new with no protection, as if I just stepped out of an egg. But I also feel open to guidance. I had a dream that behind the house was a geyser pumping Light. I need to find ways to be aware of the Light source that is there constantly. In another dream I am walking down a long hallway. I start to feel weak and crumple at the door of Swami SP's room. Someone comes and picks me up. It is a warning not to approach things in an old way.

Mataji continues to be in pain and I drive to Spokane to see her. She is now asking people to *pranam* on entering or leaving, as a way to show respect. She says the problem is lack of awareness. People put themselves first. I ask her how we can learn to think of others. And she says to practise by using a person as a representation of the Divine, then treat them as the Divine, not as the person. The temptation is for everyone to do their own thing and not follow the Divine law, not be truly human, not be willing to pay the price. They want to do it the easy way. She is also trying to wake us up by changing phrases that have become standard and mechanical. Instead of saying "Mataji," she is asking us to call her "Swami Radha." She doesn't want words to become meaningless.

"The residents need to learn to respect you too," she says. "As president, what would you like from others?" She wants me to consider protocol. She also suggests that the residents gather together to work on our dreams. Dreams are the path given by the Divine and develop intimacy with the Divine. How to instill the connection that people are precious?

When I get back to the Ashram there is a message from Swami Radha saying that she wished I could have stayed another day. She appreciated me coming down. I am humbled, feeling I have done nothing to deserve her appreciation.

I receive more news from Spokane. Susan, who was assisting Swami Radha through her illness, is leaving to be with her mother in Vancouver. I am shocked. How could she even think of abandoning her now? Swami Radha says that she is terminating their association. Susan – my longtime friend who introduced me to the teachings! How can anyone be liberated in one lifetime when there are so many traps? Susan calls me, sobbing, wanting to come to the Ashram. But it doesn't seem like the right time. She is such a symbol for people and she is so unclear in her commitment. I put the Ashram first. I put the guru first, as I have many times before, because she is my first and foremost friend.

I am personally finding inspiration through study of the original Kundalini texts and *Ananda Lahari*,[1] a scripture that honours the goddess. I read each verse and reflect on how the ancient words are present in this moment of my life. The beauty of the teachings is like an altar of flowers, available to everyone. Commitment and devotion seem to be missing ingredients in many people's lives. Why? One of the women said that I can get to the essence of something easily. I go to Divine Mother's feet, and think of Her. Is that devotion? For me devotion has been the cure, and asking questions the way to reach deep and bring up the nectar that satisfies people.

Winter 1994

At the annual general meeting a huge circle of people has gathered. As we listen to the reports I realize that the changes

---

1   Sri Sankaracharya, translation and commentary by Swami Sivananda, *Ananda Lahari: The Blissful Wave* (Calcutta: The S.P. League, 1949).

in the Ashram this year have gone at a rapid pace – with the new Mandala House underway, the new dream book[2] ready for publication, increasing enrolments all summer, and new programs being launched, including the teacher training courses and the Youth Program, which is bringing in vitality and new life.

"The transformation had to happen," Mataji told me. She knew it would put the pressure on but that is how we develop. It seems the first year needed a boost to get everything going. I am personally moving from being in a busy, tight mode to being in a busy, expansive mode. "Swami Radhananda" is a new but powerful self-image. Going through the fire means burning through the obstacles, being tested and purified, clearing the way so I can continue. Some people have left their commitments but the work and the teachings will go on.

The sound in our group changes from talk to mantra as we repeat the Light mantra, a moment when everyone has one focus – on being here. I see the approach the Light takes, bringing us to this point, this focus. I hear conviction in my voice as I draw the people close, a feeling of connection. The purpose of this group is to return to the Light. I see the space as a pool of Light with us reflected in it, influenced.

Gratitude to Swami Radha. Pressure is producing results.

---

2   Swami Sivananda Radha, *Realities of the Dreaming Mind: The Practice of Dream Yoga* (Spokane, WA: Timeless Books, 1994).

Radha Calling to Krishna

Winter 1995

In the dark night of the New Year we gather on the beach to launch small candlelit boats onto the lake, observing their progress as symbolic for our path this year. My little blue boat stays right behind the large guru boat, following her toward the sparkling lights on the other shore. Then her boat turns a corner and is out of sight.

I've been reading Swami Radha's old letters, getting a feel for how she was when she first came back from India in 1956. She was ordinary, chatty, loving, brave, trying things out, determined. Signs that she was the guru were present through how people were attracted to her – always writing to her and going out of their way to meet with her.

Swami Radha calls to say she has the Light back in the diamond ring and I can have it or keep the "pearl of great price." She wants me to know that I represent her at the Ashram. I feel humbled. I tell her that last year was a testing time for me, and now I am gaining self-confidence and respect from others. She tells me that Julie is back with her, doing well and working hard.

My days are full with board meetings, resident meetings,

groups, office activities and the launch of the new YDC. A lot is stirred up at the Ashram with the ongoing changes and more to come. Today I rearrange the Temple and reflect on what I'm observing with people – attractions, ambitions, jealousies. What is an ashram? How did Swami Radha meet all these people? In the evenings I do practices that sustain me – breath and Light, mantra, *mahamudra*, the Divine Mother prayer, Headstand, Shoulderstand, reflections on *Ananda Lahari*.

In the YDC, which is a large group of women this year, we start working with Kundalini. Women can be terrifying in their confusion and lack of love in their lives. The stories go on – their needs and dependencies and the price they've paid – abandoned children, children taken away, physical, sexual and emotional abuse. They have forgotten their true love. Yesterday I said to myself that I can handle the emotions, and today I do.

At the resident meeting after supper I look around at the group and see a certain immaturity and a continued need for training. Now I understand the idea of taking on the burden of the Ashram. Love is in helping with the burdens. I don't have the guru experience of "going beyond" to carry me through, but if love is surrender, then maybe I can do it. I trust Swami Radha but there are so few of us left here, with residents going back and forth to Spokane. We are keeping our commitment of saying "yes" to what she asks, and it is putting us under pressure. But I know it will all work out.

Today, February 2nd, we send a card and flowers for Swami Radha on her *sanyas* day. I reflect on my initiation into *sanyas* a year ago. I feel happiness throughout the day, real happiness. Last year the Temple was reserved for my initiation. Today I'm in my silk sari by 7 a.m., walking to the Temple to honour the initiation. It's dark but very warm and springlike.

Alone in the Temple I chant the mantra with conviction. I am convinced that Swami Radha was here helping me through this last year and that her trust was also a force in my initiation. I notice the spirit of what I've done, the victories, the positive workings, the determination. It starts with saying, "I can do it." "I will." Willingness. I must bring in that spirit so that behind the action is the conviction, the determination, the love, and the willingness to surrender.

I chant wholeheartedly, like Radha calling to Krishna, allowing her to have a voice.

Swami Radha's conviction is based on her own experience. Reading her history I could see that she was able to withstand the challenges of the academics, the psychologists, the '60s hippies, the malcontents, the critics, the disciples who left. She knows within herself the connection to the Divine, and that is all that counts.

A year ago at the initiation I came as I was and changed to who I am. I feel as though I have placed myself on the fire of love, been cremated, emerged new, clear, empty of old concepts, ideas burned up and with a new willingness to surrender. Surrender is love; otherwise, how could I do it? What survives is the emptiness.

I am emptying the contents of my mind for the Light, opening my heart for the action. What needs to survive? Wholeness, holiness, a holy place for worship. "Worship" is the word I chose for this New Year. I placed the word beside Swami Radha's picture on my altar as a reminder to worship as she does, to worship in the place of love.

I am empty to be filled. Initiation is a start. Rings are reminders of the promise.

In the afternoon everyone gathers for a *puja* in the Temple. I explain that the ritual is to be held in the heart and is a way to understand the deep in the drop. We chant.

with devotion, then *pranam* and offer flowers before the big pictures of Swami Radha and Swami Sivananda. When we stop chanting I hear Swami Radha's voice continuing in the silence. We eat the little oranges from the orange tree now inside the Temple. People are touched. Everything feels real, involved, not static. We dismantle the flower offerings and carry them to the lake and throw them in with abandon.

Back in class I am leading the workshop on the mind. I talk in my mind to Swami Radha, asking, What next? The students are watching their minds and I am watching them, observing inside and outside of myself. Watching my mind, observing the influences. How to approach the mind? Mind – the last frontier. Silence is all around me. I have space to think. Everything looks more level when quiet and concentrated, exploring like a landscape the inner view. I interview the mind. Who are you? Where are you? What will we do? Then I go to a knowing place. What is next becomes obvious as I get to know my own mind.

I have a few days off from teaching and drive to Spokane to be with Swami Radha. We are having a quiet time together. I am sitting across from her at her big desk when she says, "I have something for you," and she slides a little blue box across the desk. I open it and inside is the pearl tree – a lovely gold brooch with pearls as its fruit. It's a glowing moment. I know she has worn this brooch, that it has been hers. And I know there is something vast behind it, a responsibility that comes with the gift.

Swami Radha has often told the story of Krishna sending a messenger to Radha to ask for a bead of her mala so he can grow a pearl tree. Radha is very impatient, saying no one can grow a tree from a pearl and sends the messenger away. But he comes again and again until Radha finally relents, passionately saying, "I won't destroy my mala. Give him the whole thing!" The messenger takes the mala and disappears. Radha remains petulant and unbelieving until the messenger returns and leads her to a sacred grove where the tree has grown and is luminous with pearls.

When Swami Radha received this brooch as a gift she took it as a confirmation that her work and the teachings would grow and bear fruit. This pearl tree, which is being given to me, belongs to Radha. She has to share what she knows so it can bear fruit.

Swami Radha asks, "How many pearls are on it?"

I count them up. "Around thirty."

"Do you know what they represent?"

I do know. I have heard her say it many times. "Initiations."

"Thirty initiations. Choose them wisely."

I am holding this tiny precious thing. It is a confirmation about preparing to initiate others. I wonder how it will happen.

She tells me that people should *pranam* to me at the *puja*s. When they do I should touch their heads and say, *Om Namah Sivaya*. I should sit on a chair near the altar and have an extra chair, representing her on the other side of the altar. She is giving me these instructions as a way to start. She is initiating me into initiating. This is the first step, to sit at the front representing the teachings, with people bowing down before me as a symbol of Radha. I understand she wants me to take on the responsibility fully.

Later, when I am alone, I reflect on her gift. She is putting deep trust in me. I know that her warning to make my choices wisely is based on her own experience. Many people she initiated did not stay with their commitment. She hoped that this eternal bond to the mantra would be there for them. The promise of a guru is to keep coming back, lifetime after lifetime, until the disciple is liberated. She does not want to keep coming back for people who don't even make contact with her on a human level.

I will continue to share what I have been given. I know there is "something more," the power of the lineage, that will come in to help. My motivation is only to help people, even though they may not understand fully what they are getting into.

In the morning I wake up and find my hands in *namaste*, seeking the Divine in myself, seeking the Divine in others. In the soft morning glow, I see the pearl tree bearing fruits from the mantra seed planted deep within. Radha gives Krishna the fruits, affirming her willingness to grow into Light.

Will this little tree grow?

Back at the Ashram I continue to feel Swami Radha's trust. It is helpful to think of myself as Radhananda in order to face what seems difficult. I represent Swami Radha, so I must change and continue to change, being able to move toward people, present her ideas and teaching, listen for her voice. Each time there is a step forward for Radhananda, my "Mary-Ann self," the very human part, gets brought forward too. She has always aspired to spiritual life – I have only to read my old papers to see that. But she is a bit dazzled by the pearls and the price. I have to keep her posted about where we are headed and the changes I want to make, to be sure she is in agreement.

Even though I feel young in the name and position, I am maturing. And in my mind it is sometimes hard to put together the old and the new, the approachable and the distance that the position creates. I do a Straight Walk to the chair and see my "Radhananda self" there. She is approachable and becomes refined and a bit more elegant in the process. She grows in wisdom and becomes lighter. This evolution seems to be what the grace of commitment is bringing to my image now.

The Bhagavad Gita says that the world is a battlefield and the real battle is within. My battlefield is right here. D. and I are sitting beside each other, leading the Gita class. What is it that happens to my mind? What makes it difficult for us to work together on one paper or to respond harmoniously? Why does he leave the room to do the Light or redo what I say? He is a *gurubhai*, a *sanyasin*, a friend. We can usually talk about almost anything. But when we are in class, why is there an underlying battle?

He does his professional interview technique of drawing the students out and keeping track of what they say. I do things differently – allowing space, trusting their intelligence, keeping them in the Light. But when we're together I feel hesitant, trying to think as he does. Where is my conviction? How do I listen and respond?

It doesn't matter who is right or wrong, but I feel we are not connected. I see myself always in the shadow of his shoulder or side, put to one side. He is so much bigger than me and it feels like the unspoken law in the battle, that men rule and need space. I feel trapped, not able to get to what holds me back. Why can't I work with him? Do I need his approval?

I go back to my name, Radhananda, to the real part of me, the knowing part. Beyond feeling to knowing. Accept who I am. Be courageous, guided from within. I think about how I can read each student by responding to the signs my senses pick up. Then the message comes, not from any hard and fast idea or isolated facts, but through an opening to what the person presents.

What stops this ease from happening when we are together? Are we in competition? Is it the old conditioning of male and female playing out? I have to remember my duty and go straight to Radha without being clouded by subtle messages of "I can't."

I need to address this problem in a clear way – not blaming but inquiring. I also see the conflict as an internal reflection. I need to stand up to what is within myself that grabs my voice and mind space and doesn't allow the wisdom to come out. What is it that brings the tentativeness, the feeling of being diminished?

I focus on breath, settle into myself and become clear.

There is a plan to videotape an interview about me becoming the president of the Ashram. I go down to the studio and see Russell and D. preparing. Russell is operating the camera. He moves close and shows me how and where to sit, where to look and how to be. I feel as though he hovers, trying to capture me. D. interrupts to explain the interview process and suggest questions and even some anticipated responses. I feel as though they are both moving too close, corraling me, telling me what to do and say. I am also in the middle of something between the two of them.

The interview starts. I feel pressured to be someone I'm not, and I react.

"Stop!"

Something has happened and I need to see it on video. What I see is myself in relationship to this large man. I am the emotional little woman, being put down. There's even a moment where D. hits my arm jokingly, but it still hurts. It's over for me. I leave. Where is the respect? I have a voice. I know what I need to say. I cannot become their image of me.

Maybe I made it all up. I ask D. what he thought was

happening. He says when there are two men and one woman, the men always fight over the woman. He and Russell were competing for my attention. I listen but my discomfort doesn't go away.

I meet with him again later and tell him how I was feeling. He says he didn't experience anything like what I described. He is upset that I don't trust him and cuts me off, saying, "We can't work together then!" I feel as though my experience means nothing and that the familiarity between us does breed contempt. Swami Radha spoke to me about respect and then this situation comes along. I feel put down, not listened to and not trusted either.

I ask myself questions about male and female. I need to keep some distance now and if feelings arise, speak them. Even if I'm afraid, I can't let this happen. I can't lose my voice or enter into some kind of competition – over what? Power? Can they even accept that I am the president of the Ashram?

At satsang my mind brings up an old image of my mother and father, giving me a clue. I never wanted to be in a relationship like theirs – he showed no respect for her through his silence, his lack of facial expressions. She – laughing, emotional and friendly – put up with him and his other interests, work, women.

Why can't men listen to women? Why do they want to dominate? It makes it hard. Where to insist on respect, as Swami Radha does? And how do I come from the strong Radha place in myself instead of reverting to an old personality?

But even as I act, there is a witness to my activities, an aspect that is above it all. I remember the last visit with Swami Radha when she gave me the pearl tree to symbolize the initiations. It opened up something vast and luminous in me. I need to step into that Light. I also need to set some goals so my personality aspects don't interfere.

On one level, the Light is here and is vast. On the human level, I keep learning and clearing the way.

Spring 1995

Morning in the Temple is quiet, light, fresh, peaceful – like a separate world of silence. The sky is silver-blue and the lake reflects that lightness so that the world could be turned upside down and it would look the same. It's like an ancient place of beginnings. Morning light comes in long fingers across the rug. Mantra refreshes me. Thoughts have come and gone but the mantra lingers in the air.

I notice the roses on the altar for today's Rose Ceremony, marking the end of the YDC. Like the rose blossom, attraction is essential – attraction to the Divine.

I am making a space for the Divine to come in but not exposing that centre to all. Reflecting on *sanyas*, I am learning how not to control. I am learning that it is Her world, not mine, the world of Light. The Light represents a power, a source that nourishes the inner and outer selves. I remember Swami Radha saying, "I will share with you all I know. You will keep the teachings alive. Promise." Sweetness, a taste that lingers.

As a group we are holding together, doing the Light together, not self-absorbed. Everyone contributes, knowing what we need to know and setting it into action.

The Temple is filled with Light, mantra and the songs of spring birds.

I am observing my interactions with men. In what ways do I feel afraid or not trust that I have power? What limitations do I put on myself and then project out to men? I am teaching the Kundalini and Dream training courses by myself, a place of working with minds where I feel confident.

What would it mean to be placed here under the guidance of a bodhisattva? I see how in this position the learning happens, the changes occur. Crystal-clear images arise of my past, my nature, the choices I have made. I want some understanding of my life to this point.

But this is the point where my life is, and the understanding arises of now. I have no immunity. What arises needs to be dealt with. Spring – the season of redemption and resurrection. What about my response to the video? I have to look at these parts of me in the clear light, to learn about my nature, power, energy and choice.

The video incident brought forward deep feelings. I could not assume the role of the powerless woman as I saw it being played out. It was a passing glimpse on the screen but it resurrected my parents and how I saw my mother trapped in an image. At first I didn't know how to say it – there were just wordless emotions, anger. Then I realized I could not keep an old reflection spinning. I had to say no to dependence, yes to independence. Yes to responsibility, acceptance and trust.

Things are changing. Can the line of genes spin itself out?

In the work I have done on myself I see the evidence of not being swayed, of keeping with the Light, of acting consciously rather than unconsciously. The senses can be centred on awareness instead of on obstacles.

Today Julie sits in on the course with me. She is up from Spokane for a few days. She says that she can see the passion of the teachings coming through me – the passion of Radha – the same quality Swami Radha has, and it inspires her to move toward *sanyas*.

I travel to Toronto and Ottawa, leaving the Ashram and going out into the world, taking the teachings with me. At the workshops people are coming to receive. I am refocused for a purpose, toward my duty. I am becoming more myself, more relaxed. The intensity of beauty on a spring day – what is blossoming within me? The Buddha stands with the gesture of "have no fear" and says "you will be given what you need." I'm coming to see that on many levels. I'm less able to control, less wanting to control, and more able to work with what comes. The prayer wheel turns.

Returning to the Ashram I start preparing for the summer. Love is what we need for the summer, the kind that Swami Radha has to give – unending, ongoing, constant, beautiful, challenging – for each other, for ourselves and for our guests. Where does the focus and energy come from to do more? Let Krishna drive the chariot. Keep the mind on Radha. Each person can present the Light to our guests through interest, questions and approach. This will give a constant sense that they are in the Light. But we have to know and feel the gratitude ourselves first, not let it get stuffed down with busyness, upsets and misunderstandings. Set aside our limitations and use the energy to work.

How to operate the Ashram and the summer program with so few teachers here? Many of the teachers are with Swami Radha, working on her video and biography. Three residents here are going to a psychiatrist and are on Prozac. This phase won't last forever. Somehow it will change and we will be able to manage.

But first I have to go to New York City.

This year Swami Radha published her book on dreams, *Realities of the Dreaming Mind*,[1] and received an invitation to present at a dream conference in New York in June. She

---

1   Swami Sivananda Radha, *Realities of the Dreaming Mind*.

has asked her publisher and me to do the presentation for her. For the past few months I've been reviewing my dreams, gathering examples of how my dreams have guided my path. It is exciting to see how my unconscious knew more than "I" did. The work has been very rewarding but it's intimidating to imagine myself presenting it to a conference of academics in New York. I've never even been there and it's a big stretch from the Ashram.

In Spokane my colleague and I coordinate the two parts of our speech – my personal reflections with her overview of Dream Yoga. Swami Radha asks us to run through our presentation in front of her. As we practise she makes suggestions for how to improve. She wants us to be more dynamic and engaging, to feel what we are saying and project it, to look up and out at the audience. It is nerve-wracking, but she hugs us afterward and tells us how well we have done. "Let Divine Mother speak through you," she says.

In New York – stumbling onto the train with our luggage. Noise, smell, traffic, people, streets, friendliness, heat. We settle into our room and then walk around, connecting to Divine Mother in the cathedrals. We drop into the conference hall. The registrars are surprised that "the swamis" are women!

On the day of our speech we wear our saris. I am able to look out at the audience and I encourage them to use dreams to contact the spiritual reality in their lives, to access their own inner knowledge. I speak from my personal experience, which seems different from the academic approach most presenters are offering. I describe my arrival at the Ashram so many years ago, and how I recognized the cedar lodge, the creek and the cabin from a dream that I had had the night before. It was like a confirmation that I was on the right path. I describe the power line dream, and how it reassured me that the support for my position as president of the Ashram was there through this lineage that went back to the source.

And I say how each dream is like a diamond with many facets sparkling with an inner fire. The insights can lead us to a sense of wonder at the beauty and care of the path laid out before us. As I talk I am amazed that I'm not nervous. Many women gather around us afterward to ask questions.

My colleague continues to travel, and I fly back to Spokane and tell Swami Radha everything. She seems so proud of me, and she expresses it in her special way. She gives me a beautiful pearl choker with a clasp loaded with jewels – sapphires, diamonds and I don't even know all the gems – which she had received as a gift. "When you wear it," she says, "keep it hidden under a scarf. Think of it as your secret gift from Krishna, a reminder of how precious you are. Think of yourself always as Radha, cosmic love."

I wake up with a dream that Swami Radha is giving me her clothes. I wonder how I can wear them all. She is going to die, it seems.

Any More Questions?

Summer 1995

Literally being up front in the Temple, making myself public, I receive both the jealousy and the adoration, the ups and the downs. It is evident that it isn't me or mine. I'm freeing myself from control, of having my way. It's impossible anyway. What is possible is to let others do their work and gain trust by observing what comes back. No interference, which is what is happening and working for me. The pressures of the work make it possible to allow something else to come through. The work does the work.

What is it that people need? Swami Radha always gives encouragement in little ways, recognizing sincerity and effort. I need both the courage to support and the courage to be direct. I'm learning the administrative part of the Ashram, and I'm also bringing forth a motherly, loving part – Radha. What is attractive to her? Sincerity and loyalty.

How did Swami Radha awaken me? Remembering me, spending bits of time with me, loving me. How? Through straight talks, gifts, trust, giving me what was most precious – her insights, directing and supporting me, not physically but on another level. Can I access that now with others?

I am upset by Don G. He says I look burdened. I could see all week that he was trying to help women by counseling them. He is not able to hear me. I am frustrated by the way he puts me aside and runs the Ashram. In the board meeting D. says the exact same thing that I just said, and Don G. hears him but not me. It happens again with Don N., the other man on the board. I am frustrated with all the times that men can hear other men, but not women. The respect issue with men keeps coming up. What to do next?

Before supper I go for a walk, and stop to pull knapweed, a noxious invasive weed, by the Temple. Don G. comes out of the Temple and invites me in. He says a woman from the course has something to tell me. "Thank you for protecting the Ashram!" she says. "It's so wonderful to be in this safe place for women." Such a message – arising, it seems, almost from the voice of the Temple!

This morning Don G. comes over and says, "I wonder why I couldn't hear you yesterday when you said the same thing as D.? I am perplexed." I said I was too. He asks if he can sit in on my next meeting so he can learn.

My thoughts go to evolution again. Do we hold each other back or can we grow toward the Light?

Swami Radha has asked Don G. to attend a *bandhara* in Berkeley, to find out how they do it. A *bandhara* is a celebration of a guru's life, literally meaning "opening the storehouse." It happens when the guru passes on.

I am doing the Headstand in the middle of my room

– seven times today. This was a hard pose for me to achieve, but now I can do it freestanding and I feel this strong desire to turn my world upside down. How can I take an opposite view and challenge my thinking?

Kundalini teacher training is launched and leads people to their innermost selves. The ashram group is stretched, with two more people in Spokane. There is a growing group of young people here that seem like a new beginning. They are not stuck in rules, and they bring joy, freshness and willingness to come right in and help. I'm turning my world upside down, letting go of the old ways and opening to the new …

Swami Radha has had a big change of heart too. Up until now, she has given mantra initiations only to students she has known for many years, those who have been close to her and gained her confidence by their commitment and sincerity. But now she has announced that she will be giving a mantra pronouncement on September 8th, her guru's birthday, and that anyone who wants to receive the mantra can come.

Some of the people here and at the Radha Centres have been hoping for initiation from Swami Radha for years, but she was firm that the opportunity was over and the door was closed. Now she is opening it up again, following Gurudev's tradition of throwing out the seeds to grow where they will. It will be up to each person whether or not they nurture this seed.

She also tells me privately that she is giving me more time to get ready.

Arriving in Spokane I see Swami Radha and feel her presence as Light. She seems particularly luminous, even as her body becomes tinier and more fragile. She tells me that she keeps me in her mind, knowing the difficulties of the Ashram. She asks me to arrange a time after the mantra pronouncement to meet with the young people. My children, Garth and Clea, have decided to come and receive the mantra from her. I feel joyful for them.

"How will the mantra pronouncement work?" I ask her.

"One mantra," she says, "with many people. It's open to all. You can even ask your mother to come. Anyone who is in the building will benefit."

Swami Radha tells of her plans for a spiritual marriage for Deborah and Charles, an ashram couple who have been working with her on the video biography. She says it will be a private event to help them sustain each other and bring quality to their marriage. She asks me to conduct the ceremony.

In the afternoon I prepare the altar, and in the evening I lead them in a Rose Ceremony. They read their commitment papers to each other. I ask them to reflect on qualities that attracted them to the other and to bring out those same qualities in themselves. Afterward we go to Swami Radha's apartment. She puts on lively Indian music and encourages us all to dance. It's a festive occasion, and she is radiant and very happy.

"As the president of the Ashram," Swami Radha says, "you deserve a special status at the mantra pronouncement. I want to show my respect for you. How should I incorporate you?" I am so surprised, that she, of all people, would be concerned about respecting me; I am her disciple. But she says I am more than that. She will have the speaker introduce me as the Ashram's president and I can give the welcoming introduction.

September 8, 1995. One hundred and forty people have gathered from everywhere. I welcome them, and together we chant.

We are coming together to bring out the sacredness and live it, a commitment. The commitment is to the security and insecurity of the mantra, to listen to it, to surrender to it, to bring it to life, to build trust in the sacred words. Trust, a blessing. Being infused with mantra, letting the stillness and quiet be filled with sacred sound, we prepare for the blessing, being together in support. This sound has a place to live in my heart.

Swami Radha enters and the chanting continues. She stops and the silence resonates with vibration. Out of the silence, her voice firm and clear pronounces, "*Hari Om.*"

As the chanting resumes she is there, being able to give to each person as they come up and offer her a gift and their mala to be blessed. Even if they are far away, she reaches out and gives them what she can. The flow never stops – the flow of people up to her and the flow of the mantra through her. She is the vessel, yet very present in this world, conscious of each person, each gift, each mala. It is amazing to see her become an overflowing fountain of Light.

The day after the mantra pronouncement, she talks with Garth and Clea about the difficulties of life in this time of multinational corporations and lack of care for the individual. She encourages them to find their own path. At my initiation she had asked what was most precious to me, and I said my children. I knew she would look after them at a different level. And she has.

Fall 1995

At the Ashram the moon is stamped on the morning sky, a seal that the night has passed. I'm talking to Don G. about attraction. What people love and how they love can be turned into an approach to the teacher.

In the summer there was so much work and busyness, so many people. Now in the fall there is stillness. It is all part of the harmony. Accepting the rhythms of life, working with the harmony – mind blends the elements of time and space, solid and ethereal, mind and body, action and thought. What is the work? Swami Radha is encouraging me to do a different kind of work – to study, reflect and wonder. I am learning to let go of the need to always be active.

What if I am responsible to the Divine for the people here? What would that mean? Humility is part of it. Doing what I am asked to do. What is an ashram? Could we get bogged down in bureaucracy, or in thinking we are a family and getting all tied up with each other instead of learning to trust the Divine? Has the Divine been wrong yet? What is a mistake then? What is fear of making a mistake?

In the afternoons we gather together for work bees, enjoying the gifts of the season. Today we are juicing apples – golden, rich, very sweet juice, streaming, steaming. The fall weather is crisp warm, bright, liquid honey light. What is harmony? Being present, working together. It reminds me of the red line that ran through one of my drawings in a Music and Consciousness workshop years ago, up and down through the whole piece. How do we find our way? Through talking, asking questions, not knowing. Still the apples ripen, the work needs to be done and we do it.

Can anyone really do it "my way" or is that only a longer way? I'm staying with the process – using the Light, being receptive. My direction is to practise patience with people. Patience equals love.

Swami Radha says to make sure, as president, that I don't focus just on what I want to have done, but that I really think deeply about people, events and the Ashram. Not to push.

Coming from a family of eight children, my mind is practised at managing, scheming, maneuvering. I need to go to another place. This summer I could see where I wanted it to be my way, but it simply wasn't possible. I wanted to have more experienced teachers and workers, but we were a small group. We worked with who was there and everyone benefited. Newer teachers gained more confidence and young people moved into responsible positions. The only way I could bring about change was by accepting what is and being creative within the limitations of people and time.

We need to take this opportunity to be here seriously and address issues and see clearly what we have to do. We need to work with a purpose and use the time wisely. We're not here forever.

I dream that we are moving to a new location. Start small.

It is the first day of a new discipline. We start at 6 a.m. with chanting in the Temple. Everyone arrives five minutes early and we walk in together. In the evening we all meet again and walk in together for satsang. Our practice is to be together as a group in order to gain strength. We are also committing to respecting time by arriving early – for chanting, for satsang and for all of our meals. It is a small beginning but everyone seems slightly ecstatic. People are putting forth their best effort. We will emerge solid, knowing and capable.

L. has come back to Canada from Mexico for a visit to her family and friends. But instead of returning as planned she has decided to leave the work altogether and to give up her commitment. She is here at the Ashram packing up all her stuff. Her wedding ring is back on her finger and she does not want to meet with us.

Each week now we practise Aikido. Swami Radha wanted us to learn a martial art to become stronger and to learn to hold our ground. Aikido has taught me to enter the space and go with the roll when I'm thrown – a technique I'm getting better at applying in my life. It has been a year of many leavings and I'm rolling with them.

Some people are here but they start to leave in their minds. I find it sad when the connection to the work is not strong enough to go beyond sentiment to steadiness and strength. I often see a desire for people to have their way. Pride. What do people do in order to be liked? How far would they go? Some have the tendency to leave.

My job now is to stay connected, to enter the heart, to build that space like a temple within myself. I am on the front line and am willing to be there for Swami Radha, so she can do whatever she needs to. She passes the techniques to me, step by step. I learn from the meetings with people and the leavings. I take the roll, enter the space, be aware of the spiritual energy, not just my own little reaction. Let it come in and let it go. Divine Mother weeds her garden.

The lineage is a connection built on faith and the path of Light, step by step. The support is behind me. I know a connection has been made, unbroken, eternal.

I make a quick, unexpected trip to Spokane. Swami Radha seems well and happy. She asks how my kids are after the mantra pronouncement and she talks about the temptation to train young people for the Ashram. "They must experience life first," she says, "otherwise it would not be for their benefit." She wants to know how everyone is doing at the Ashram, and we talk about which residents should come down next to check in with her. I don't know how she decides or who she needs to see. Sometimes it seems as if most of the Ashram is here.

How hard it is to surrender to that! But I always remember our promise to say "yes," and I know that each person gains so much from her care. She also reminds me that I have much more support than she ever had. She is so right!

A phrase resounds in my head from the visit with her, "I can give you the money now for the Mandala House project," as if I were the Ashram. She shows her support for our projects in such tangible ways. Many people feel most comfortable donating directly to her, and she passes the donations on to support the expanding work.

I will have been at the Ashram five years this December. I've started a diary review to see what I have learned in this time. The challenge has been to understand the power of words and also the power of love. Love means to be secure in the Light, not to be attached to my ideas or concepts. Attachments give me a limited view of others and myself. Love, or the expression of the Light, brings fullness. I am letting go of people's ideas of me, too.

How did I start on this spiritual path? What seeds of potential were already there? My life seemed very ordinary. Growing up in the '50s, I had limited career opportunities as a woman, so I took up teaching. How does the energy live within the confines of work, marriage, family, friends, environment? Was there always direction? Only when I became aware could I expand the meaning of my life. I think the sincerity of wanting to help Swami Radha was the basis for my development.

I return daily to the Temple now. I need time alone. In my first years at the Ashram I was in the Temple each evening. Now I am letting Divine Mother lead me back. I go to the Temple and fill my mind with the sound of mantra. The response comes in the moment of silence when I can listen.

My practice is to have the humility to listen – to Divine
Mother, to other people. Whenever I am with someone, first I
listen to what they have to say. Then I surrender to the power
of love in whatever person She sends me.

The Divine Mother prayer makes Her come alive. My
concerns about people fade. It's as if She sits at my elbow,
holding me gently, loosely. When I concentrate on Her,
letting Her work through me, I feel lifted up physically and
mentally by Her Light – supported, receptive to the Light but
willing to take action and speak about what I hear.

Sometimes I feel I could go into silence easily. But then
I'm faced with a person who is stuck, and I have the desire
to reach out and help them move beyond it. Five years ago I
needed to ask questions. Now I need to ask questions. I also
need to gather my discoveries. If I ignore what I've learned,
I'm not listening to Her.

I see there is a power in the Light that reveals what is
going on. Looking back over the past five years I can see I
know more about myself and I've put some things aside,
but I am essentially me. I have seen others struggle and their
divinity arise up out of the ashes. Each rising is different, each
path unique.

Mine is a joyous journey of exploration, looking at facts
and feelings, balancing the opposites and coming to centre in
stillness. I'm coming to centre in the movement storm, not
affected by the polarities, focusing on Her.

November 18–22, 1995

Swami Radha has asked Don G. and me to come to Spokane
and spend time with her. We bring our questions about
ashram situations, specific people, money, policies and where
we are at, so that she can comment and give us guidance.

She is interested in everything – how we think, how we visualize the future, how we deal with the immediate issues that need clarification. She tells us how she has handled similar situations in the past. She talks about the obstacles and strengths in her different disciples. And she tells us why she has shaped the Ashram's guiding principles in the way she has.

But her main message is this: "Do the work as your personal service to the Divine."

And she asks, "What is your supreme offering to the Divine?" What can we actually do, remake, develop or overcome that would make our lives a supreme offering? She says people tell her that they have offered their lives, but they do not make any sacrifices.

"What is your supreme offering?"

I think of the story she tells of Ramakrishna holding a man's head under water and telling him that he can come back when he wants the teachings as badly as he wants to breathe. I am willing to do whatever has to be done. I am willing to sacrifice comfort, control, whatever I am aware of as an obstacle. I call on sincerity.

Her desire for me is to understand, and my desire is to understand her. She offers assurance. "You will always have my complete support. I am behind you one hundred percent."

I notice she is eating practically nothing. What is supporting her body? She is this transparent being, overflowing with Light, sitting day and night trying to find ways to bring people in. She quenches the thirst of those who come close. Some drink it up and become part of the flow. Some don't like what she offers and reject it. Others remain in dryness.

After hours of long meetings she laughs and says the real reason I'm here is to file her fingernails. I move in close to her, doing something simple with her body, connecting to her Light.

On our last day in Spokane a group of us gather together with her. She says, "I am very happy to see how the Ashram is functioning now. I can say goodbye with a happy heart." She looks at me intently and asks, "Do you have any more questions? Is there anything else you need to know?"

I pause, thinking back to our meetings over the past five days. "No, you have answered all our questions. Thank you. You've given us so much!"

Back at the Ashram, I reflect on our time together. I remember a vision from a few years ago of Swami Radha asking if I will help. I promise I will. I promise I will not forget her. This elusive ideal of remembering also means to remember a knowing part in myself and to trust it. What can I do to discover that other world I know is there? How do I step into it, leave this shore and plunge into the ocean of Light?

November 30, 1995

I receive a call from Spokane that Swami Radha has passed into the Light. She is gone. Is it possible? I think of her words, "Do you have any more questions?"

Love Love Love

We drive the van down to Spokane to return her body
to the Ashram. She looks peaceful, almost as though she
is breathing. I do the Light for her essence, but I feel the
blessing is really mine. I know she was joyous and victorious
and went quickly to the Light. She is Radha, and Krishna's
arms were waiting for her, her job complete.

In my mind I tell her that people at the Ashram are
preparing her room in readiness. They are following her
instructions to decorate the four-poster bed with garlands
and to clear the way around the bed so that people can say
their last goodbyes. She was always very private, but she
was still willing to make this final sacrifice to fulfill her
disciples' needs.

I wonder how I will carry on. But I have been in this
position for a while, so I will keep going the same way. There
will be the same sense of knowing it is right action when I feel
connected to her. What are the powers she has given me? Her
trust, the power to teach in her name, allowing me to know
her. Her love.

Driving back we do everything with care, aware of the

preciousness of her body. As we cross the border a double rainbow appears, and in Creston we find bouquets of fresh orchids, her favourite flowers. At the Ashram there are phone calls to make. People are coming from everywhere.

Radha is dissolving back into cosmic form. That is why she had the goddess name. Goddesses are larger than life. I have a knowing that there is more, and that she is here in the mantra, given and received. Her expansive nature comes through. Love. Everything reminds me of her and how she has shown love.

Love, love, love.

We keep the whole week in her spirit. She asked that the service be joyful, not gloomy. The Temple is full of sunlight. People are gathered from around the world. I wear the blue silk sari from my initiation. We light candles and pass the Light to others, seeing the preciousness of each person. The sun travels up my back, warming it. I say the words for her, feeling very young and tentative, but doing my best. Everywhere there is Light.

She died as she lived her life, knowing her time, knowing the signs. As we enter the Sun Room after the service sunlight shines in and little rainbows from the crystals in the window dance on the floor, on the bed, on her body. We walk around her four-poster bed in the beauty of the room. She is wearing a simple white gown made for this purpose. I have the feeling that her death is what she always described it as – her wedding with Krishna, her reunion with the Divine.

We have dinner at the new Mandala House, which is almost completed. The residents and swamis serve the guests, in the spirit of sharing the abundance she gave us. This is the *bandhara* – the opening of the storehouse of teachings, represented by the feast. I talk about what we learned from saying "yes" to Swami Radha over the past year, and how the learning arose from pressure. I tell everyone that we intend to keep ourselves under that pressure by saying "yes" to the Divine and challenging our limitations. Everything may not be perfect at the Ashram, but we are willing, and what will emerge will be in her service.

Today is a cold day with misty wisps on the lake like vortexes of steam hovering. I glimpse an orange glow on the mountains at sunrise but it turns into a completely inward day of fog and snow. Her body is taken to the crematorium.

A year ago I was unprepared for her to die. I didn't know enough. One year, what does it bring? This last year was a stretch for me to go beyond myself to see that it is Krishna driving the chariot, and it is the Divine Source that runs the Ashram. I am given what is needed to gain strength. The ways of the Divine become evident.

My promise is to remember her. Remember her ways. Remember the involvement and inspiration. Remember the qualities and bring them to life. Learn from her unique approach, her unexpectedness, her ability to see the signs and look beyond to understanding.

I am responsible and I also know my limits. My responsibility is to look at now, to look ahead, to look over the horizon. Not everyone is supposed to live at the Ashram. It is a training ground. Let the work do the work – let it bring out what it will.

Stay together, she said. Support each other in the Light, not in the emotional gratification. The Ashram is a spiritual business. We have to run it ethically, run it in trust, let it bloom. Translate her ideals as she brought them to me. She was uncompromising about the work and the Ashram. No one or nothing is more important, yet it is through the people that the ideals are lived. They are the work. Have patience.

Trust. Trustees. Trust in the Divine. Here is the legacy,

the treasure of the teachings, her guidance and dreams.

I remember her pain and her surrender, her way of teaching us to understand. She had us come forward to do the work, going beyond ourselves to something greater.

People exclaim over my position. "It must be tremendously, incredibly demanding!" Their words are overwhelming and make me tired. Just connect with her. Speak the truth. Do. Understand the power of her words and the need to have a vehicle for them. Love will spread the word, love of the guru and a real desire to help.

I remember sitting beside her and hearing her tell stories of Gurudev.

I say, "You tell the same stories."

"Yes," she says, "because they are true."

To teach, the words need to be true, practical, liveable. Her stories arise in my mind, and the questions she asked that let me dive deeper into who I am. Words whispered, "I am so happy you are here!" Is that what the secret oral teachings are all about – love and the way to access it?

She waited patiently for everything to fall into place, for people to leave, for people to come. Let the Divine give and take away. Don't make it happen or I take on that responsibility. My responsibility is to focus on the Divine and draw from that unseen source.

As I chant today I think there has to be meaning that comes through the mantra, otherwise it is just naming the energy. But to actually enter it I have to go into depth, not just play the notes or call the name but find out what is there. Plunge into the Light. It is the same with myself. I am more than my name. I am a representative of her, not a mere surface. Look for the depth in myself – the something more.

Today is winter solstice, my fifth anniversary of being at

the Ashram. Forty years ago Swami Radha was with Gurudev at his ashram in India. I am missing her, yet knowing she is here, feeling her touch in the breeze. She is on the breath, on the mantra as it comes in and fills me. It makes it easy to remember her. It makes it hard because I know she isn't here, in that other sense.

Clearing my mind through breath and mantra, straightening my body, opening and waiting. On an in-breath, I have a vision of Swami Radha handing me a book with everything written in it. Is it the Kundalini book? The book of life? The book is tiny, like a little Bible. I exhale and turn to the next page, the next stage.

I am pleased that she could leave with a happy heart.

Resources

Yasodhara Ashram, yoga retreat and study centre
P.O. Box 9, Kootenay Bay, BC, Canada V0B 1X0
1-800-661-8711
yashram@yasodhara.org
www.yasodhara.org

International Radha Yoga Centres
www.radha.org

About the Author

Swami Radhananda is the spiritual director of Yasodhara Ashram in Kootenay Bay, BC, Canada. Appointed president of the Ashram in 1993 by her guru, Swami Radha, she carries forward the spirit of Swami Radha's work with heart, creativity and practicality.

Under her stewardship Yasodhara Ashram has thrived as a harmonious community built on the spirit of generosity and inclusion. The Ashram is also a leader in environmental sustainability.

Swami Radhananda encourages practitioners to live their yoga in daily life and to realize their potential through self-inquiry, service and devotion.

She teaches across North America and in Europe.